Health Crisis Communication

Sheng-Hsun Lee develops a new way of understanding public health crisis communication through the lens of multimodal classification. He draws on examples from COVID-19 press conferences in Taiwan and public online comments to outline multimodal classification as sorting pandemic phenomena into categorical types.

Lee argues that when public health officials classify health crisis phenomena into categories, they also set parameters for official responses and shape public perceptions of a crisis. He illustrates the argument by examining Taiwan's initial successes in keeping most infections at bay and subsequent challenges of obtaining enough vaccines for international border reopening. The successes and challenges are closely linked to multimodal classification, which includes using speech, gestures, and objects to make some categories travel broadly and impede the circulation of other categories. The book discusses a wide range of crisis categories from the three dreadful first times—the first confirmed case, the first community-acquired case, and the first death—to the politicized debate over vaccine brands. Lee emphasizes the importance of understanding how crisis categories are produced, circulated, and received. The comprehensive coverage looks beyond initial responses to the COVID-19 pandemic and outside English-dominant places to redefine effective public health messaging. Based on the findings, the book highlights implications for communicating official messages and offers a list of ready-to-use strategies for updating existing guidelines on public health communication.

The book is an essential read for public health practitioners, researchers, and advanced students in discourse analysis and public health communication.

Sheng-Hsun Lee is a Lecturer in School of Languages and Cultures at the University of Queensland. He researches health communication and language acquisition. His research has been published in international journals such as *Applied Linguistics* and *Language in Society*.

Routledge Studies in Language, Health and Culture

Series Editor: Olga Zayts

University of Hong Kong, Hong Kong

This series has several distinctive features. First, it investigates health communication through linguistic lenses. The contributions introduce the readers to a range of linguistic approaches, including, but not limited to (critical) discourse analysis, sociolinguistics, multimodal analysis, corpus analysis, and conversation analysis. Each volume draws on authentic empirical data from a range of healthcare contexts, going beyond the traditional doctor-patient encounters and expanding the focus of inquiry.

Second, the series focuses specifically on contexts outside of the mainstream English-dominant healthcare contexts, encouraging proposals from contributors working on healthcare communication in Asia-Pacific, South America, and continental Europe.

Third, some contributions focus on multicultural and multilingual healthcare encounters, thus making the series of relevance to a broad readership around the world.

The series encourages contributions that, in addition to advancing the linguistic field, also stress relevance to professional practice.

The Social Nature of Antibiotic Overprescription in China
Medical Conversations, Doctor–Patient Relationships, and Decision-Making
Nan Christine Wang

Registerial Expertise in Traditional Chinese Medical Translation
Yan Yue

Health Crisis Communication
Multimodal Classification for Pandemic Preparedness
Sheng-Hsun Lee

For more details on the series, please visit: https://www.routledge.com/Routledge-Studies-in-Language-Health-and-Culture/book-series/RSLHC

Health Crisis Communication

Multimodal Classification for Pandemic Preparedness

Sheng-Hsun Lee

Routledge
Taylor & Francis Group
LONDON AND NEW YORK

First published 2026
by Routledge
4 Park Square, Milton Park, Abingdon, Oxon OX14 4RN

and by Routledge
605 Third Avenue, New York, NY 10158

Routledge is an imprint of the Taylor & Francis Group, an informa business

British Library Cataloguing-in-Publication Data
A catalogue record for this book is available from the British Library

ISBN: 9781032898636 (hbk)
ISBN: 9781032898643 (pbk)
ISBN: 9781003545002 (ebk)

DOI: 10.4324/9781003545002

Typeset in Galliard
by Newgen Publishing UK

To Ching-Hui Wang and Jung-Hua Lee

Contents

Figures

Tables

Acknowledgements

Writing this book was not a lonely process. It involved numerous conversations online, at the office, in the classroom, and around the dinner table. At the University of Queensland (UQ), friends and colleagues in the School of Languages and Cultures provided much support and help. Guy Ramsay listened to my plan regarding a research project on multimodal communication in public health. He offered suggestions at various stages of writing this book. Valeria Sinkeviciute pointed out relevant studies about categorization when I initially mentioned my interest in studying classification. I enjoyed many inspiring conversations with her about categories and social order. Valeria and Guy took tremendous time to read the drafts of the book and offered suggestions. I am deeply grateful for their help. Melody Wei-Lin Chang listened to my ups and downs as I explored a new field of research. She generously shared her publishing experience as I assembled materials for the book. Ming-Yang Yen has been a reliable research assistant. His help with the project made data collection, transcription, and analysis less intimidating. Will Brown used her language acumen to help refine the English translation of Chinese transcripts. Stephanie Scott's copyediting always amazed me with ways of making ideas more accessible. Kayoko Hashimoto and Noriko Iwashita shared their valuable experiences of publishing books.

As I learned to present ideas in a book format, I also benefited from the exchanges with people outside my institution. Alissa Hartig and Celeste Kinginger witnessed the start of the study and the final production of the book. Along the way, they provided mental support and helpful suggestions, which have been indispensable to my research. I also would like to thank Pen-Ying Wang for her continuous support of my research by reading my research proposals, providing helpful suggestions, and creating opportunities for me to receive feedback at her institution. I am extremely indebted to her. Olga Zayts offered supportive and positive responses to my queries about publishing in the series and provided helpful comments on my proposal. Katie Peace and her team provided guidance at each book publishing stage. Two anonymous reviewers for Routledge offered incisive comments and helpful suggestions, which helped sharpen the book. I thank them for their help.

Institutional support made the completion of this book possible. It would have been very difficult to complete the book on time if it were not for a semester-long research leave from UQ in 2023. Part of the data used in the book was collected through the support of a travel fellowship from the Australian Academy of the Humanities. The fellowship not only provided financial support for data collection but more importantly, deepened my decision to study public health communication. I thank the Taiwan Centers for Disease Control for their permission to use two graphs in the book.

Finally, I must give my deepest gratitude to my parents, Ching-Hui Wang and Jung-Hua Lee, for their love and support.

Acronyms and Abbreviations

AIT	American Institute in Taiwan
BNT	BioNTech or Pfizer-BioNTech
CDC	Centers for Disease Control
CECC	Central Epidemic Command Center
DPP	Democratic Progressive Party
IDAS	Infectious Disease Announce System
ICD	International Classification of Diseases
KMT	Kuomintang, also known as Chinese Nationalist Party
LIMS	Laboratory Information Management System
MCA	Membership Categorization Analysis
PCR	Polymerase Chain Reaction
TSMC	Taiwan Semiconductor Manufacturing Company
WHO	World Health Organization

Transcription Symbols

The following conventions were adopted in transcribing and presenting interactional data in this book. For detailed descriptions of the features, see Du Bois et al. (1993).

=	lengthening
-	truncated word
--	truncated intonation unit
[ ], [[ ]], [3 3]	speech overlap
..	short pause
...	medium pause
(N)...	long pause
,	continuing
.	final
<A A>	rapid speech
<F F>	loud
<L L>	slow speech
<P P>	soft
<HI HI>	higher pitch
<RH RH>	rhythmic
<TW TW>	Taiwanese Minnan
<MRC MRC>	each word distinct and emphasized
()	vocal noise
(TSK)	click of the tongue
(THROAT)	cleaning throat
(())	transcriber comment
@	laughter
X	indecipherable syllable
Multimodality	speech co-occurred with multimodal signs

1 Introduction

1 那名台商是重症還是輕症? 從臨床判斷。
'Are the Taiwanese businessperson's symptoms severe or mild, clinically diagnosed?'[1]
2 我們今天公布的這兩個確診的案例是不是代表有社區感染?
'Do the two confirmed cases that we announced today indicate that there is community infection?'
3 我國目前的疫情大概是處於圍堵期還是已經進入了減災期?
'Is the pandemic status of our nation roughly in the containment phase, or has it already entered the mitigation phase?'

Throughout the COVID-19 pandemic, health officials in Taiwan held regular press conferences to communicate with the public about the pandemic situation and offer official responses. During those conferences, journalists often asked the officials classification questions. Such questions required the officials to explain what categories most appropriately described concepts such as virus, disease, patient, vaccine, community, and pandemic. These categories occasionally existed in pairs, as in 'severe or mild.' They also sometimes appeared in singular form, as in 'community infection.' In both formats, the journalists essentially circumscribed officials' responses by forcing the officials to explain the relationship between the categories and crisis circumstances. However, these categories were not merely descriptive labels. They also carried with them inferences and implications. For example, public fear was likely to intensify if the category 'severe' was used to describe the impact that a novel communicable disease could have on human bodies. The category 'community infection' implied that the outbreak was still controllable, but a declaration of 'community spread' across nations might have triggered the World Health Organization (WHO) to declare the virus a public health emergency of international concern and characterize the outbreak as a pandemic. Similarly, the categories 'containment' and 'mitigation' conveyed different degrees of control that the government had over the outbreak. All of this suggests that there are consequences for selecting categories from a system and using the categories to describe a person, situation, or object. At times, it can be as trivial as

DOI: 10.4324/9781003545002-1

requiring officials to elaborate on their criteria for classification. In other cases, the consequences can be as serious as a travel ban imposed by other nations or an investigation launched by the WHO, which can hurt a country's international image and economic activity. The stakes are high.

In *Health Crisis Communication*, I examine this central practice of public health communication by teasing apart the multimodal features of classification and theorizing classification in the course of crisis management. I draw on examples of COVID-19 press conferences in Taiwan to illustrate different aspects of pandemic-related classification. A research assistant and I began collecting videos of Taiwanese COVID-19 press conferences in early 2020. During the initial phase of data collection, we were not aware that we were documenting what would come to be a prolonged period of grappling with new norms and expectations. Achieving even a modicum of stability during the pandemic required constant shifting in response to the evolving pandemic situation. What worked one day could be overthrown by tomorrow's virus variant. The press conference became the epicenter of announcing and disseminating these changes. Tensions flared during the conferences, particularly between health officials and journalists, when one side saw the changes as inconsistencies but the other side regarded the changes as exigencies. Conference interaction became confrontational in the democratic society of Taiwan, where journalists have the authority to speak on behalf of the public and hold the government accountable for its opinions and actions (Clayman, 2002; Liu, 2024). During the COVID-19 pandemic, advancements in livestreaming technology on social media exposed these unsettling moments.

As we witnessed these changes, my research assistant and I kept extending our data collection plan to cover a broader time scope beyond the initial outbreak. Every time we decided to extend data collection for another year, we earnestly hoped that it would be our last extension and that life would soon return to its pre-pandemic normalcy. Yet regular COVID-19 resurgences dashed our hopes. Rather than be consumed by desperation, we turned the data collected from 2020 to 2023 into a database that we used for longitudinally tracking the ups and downs of health crisis communication. The database comprises hundreds of hours of press conference footage, millions of public online replies to the footage, and multimedia of health officials reflecting on the crisis. In retrospect, the data that we amassed are emblematic of this era of contingencies, uncertainties, and hopes, as new classifications were regularly introduced to promote official perspectives and shape the public imagination of the crisis.

This extraordinarily rich database has enabled the analysis seen here—an analysis that brings to light the intricacies of public health messaging. First, the book analyzes the multimodalities of classification. That is, it invites readers to consider the orchestration of language, gestures, placards, and eye gaze carried out by Taiwanese health officials as they crafted public health messages.

Second, the analysis engages with and expands upon the growing body of literature on COVID-19 discourse. Discourse analytical research on public health communication during COVID-19 has uncovered important language features reflecting racism (e.g., Nagar, 2023), crisis leadership (e.g., Seargeant, 2023), and pandemic framing (e.g., Charteris-Black, 2021). However, while growing scholarly attention is being paid to the initial response to the pandemic in 2020, the list of books devoted to the subsequent years of the pandemic remains short (Wallace-Wells, 2023). To understand the years that follow 2020, the analysis I provide in *Health Crisis Communication* is longitudinal in design. I consider different classifications from the start of the pandemic in 2020 to the reopening of borders by Taiwan in 2022.

Third, the book holistically captures the processes of producing, circulating, and receiving biomedical information about COVID-19, which Briggs (2024) called biocommunicability. I explore biocommunicability by triangulating my multimodal discourse analysis of press conference recordings with a content analysis of public online comments and media coverage of controversial issues about biocommunicability. My ultimate aim in writing this book is to provide practical suggestions for updating existing public health communication guidelines, which today generally prioritize the content of messages over their linguistic and multimodal construction. It is not my intent to issue a verdict on official health measures but rather to elucidate the linguistic and multimodal features that underpin crisis classification.

In what follows, I start by reviewing studies on official health crisis discourse in the fields of sociolinguistics, applied linguistics, critical discourse studies, and linguistic anthropology, all of which emphasize the importance of understanding language use in constructing public health messages. Following this review, I introduce my transdisciplinary study with four attributes that allow it to fill in the gaps in the existing research: multimodal interaction, longitudinal retracing, holistic communicability, and practical triangulation. After identifying the purpose of the study, I define and elaborate on the discursive practice of classification, which serves as the basis for my analysis in subsequent chapters. I then explain why Taiwan's pandemic experience is worthy of research attention, detail the data I have collected and used in writing this book, and account for the methods I have adopted in data analysis and triangulation. The chapter concludes with an overview and summary of the subsequent chapters.

Official Health Crisis Discourse

Much has been written about the discourse of epidemics and pandemics such as HIV/AIDS (Black, 2019; Higgins & Norton, 2010), SARS (Chiang & Duann, 2007), H1N1 (Briggs & Hallin, 2016), and COVID-19 (Jones, 2021a; Collins & Koller, 2023; Seargeant, 2023). Such studies have uncovered ways in which a communicable disease is valorized through language use. While there are wide-ranging discourses on public health, the production of knowledge by government and public health officials has continuously attracted scholarly interest.

Metaphors are commonly used by officials to provide a conceptual understanding of important social matters, including government responses to crises. Consider the example of war metaphors. In the face of a life-threatening virus, war metaphors may become propaganda tools for populist leaders of government—for example, UK Prime Minister Boris Johnson who announced his "battle plan" on the COVID-19 pandemic, and US President Donald Trump who declared himself "a wartime president"—because war metaphors not only describe what is happening but also justify actions and policies (Hanne, 2022). War metaphors also position the government and its citizens in a hierarchy, in doing so challenging representative democracy in which government representatives are elected by the public (Collins & Koller, 2023). French President Emanuel Macron had to drop war metaphors and appeal to solidarity and equality during COVID-19 after his popularity dropped significantly due to high mortality rates and overcrowded hospitals (Wodak, 2021). Indeed, the few national leaders who effectively managed the COVID-19 crisis such as the German Chancellor Angela Merkel and New Zealand Prime Minister Jacinda Ardern, avoided war metaphors and opted for other figures of speech such as "bubbles" and "thin ice" (Adams, 2020; Paulus, 2020).

Of course, there have long been conflicting opinions regarding the use of war metaphors because these metaphors in almost all uses normalize actual war, dramatize reality, surrender unlimited power to authority, and foster nationalism by inciting xenophobia (Buruma, 2020; Jenkins, 2020; Sontag, 1978). In light of these negatives about war metaphors, metaphor research stresses the importance of identifying and proposing nonmilitary metaphors for strategically communicating urgency, collaboration, and hope. A group of researchers brought this goal to fruition through an online initiative named #ReframeCovid that collected and compiled nonmilitary metaphors for reconceptualizing the COVID-19 health emergency (Olza et al., 2021).

In addition to metaphor, the scholarly literature on pandemic discourse points to the importance of narratives in constructing political leadership. Narration is a critical means by which government officials and political leaders communicate with the public during a health emergency. Stories can be used as exemplars or cautionary tales in communicating and managing a crisis, a phenomenon that Wodak (2021) called mythopoesis. However, the COVID-19 literature presents mixed results when it comes to the use of narratives by politicians. Donald Trump and Boris Johnson used illness narratives to construct their "strong leadership" and evade criticism over their failures to contain the virus (Jones, 2021b). Likewise, Boris Johnson's special advisor, Dominic Cummings, held an impromptu conference to account for his breaching of a lockdown order. Seargeant (2023) showed that Cummings's narrative account provoked controversy because the narration blended his personal life with his duty as a civil servant by using the language of emotional motivation (e.g., "I was worried ..."), causal significance (e.g., "my tentative conclusion ..."), and family identities (e.g., "leaving my wife and child at home all day and off into the night"). A lack of authenticity—i.e., driving long-distance to ensure his eyesight was not impaired by COVID-19—further undermined the credibility of Cummings's account. In contrast to other politicians, who were roundly criticized for their failures in leadership, New York Governor Andrew Cuomo effectively used narratives to enact an authentic and family-oriented persona in public, which helped him appear a trustworthy and reliable leader when communicating his stay-at-home order during the initial outbreak of the COVID-19 pandemic (Vásquez, 2021).

Leadership also emerges through other discursive practices. For instance, Jacinda Ardern successfully led New Zealand through the initial outbreak of the COVID-19 pandemic. She constructed her leadership discourse by drawing on sport metaphors that were central to collective cultural experience, skillfully maneuvering between transactional and relational talk, presenting both positive and negative visions for a possible future, and collaborating with other government officials and mainstream media (Hafner & Sun, 2021). Jacinda Ardern's example shows that the construction of crisis leadership does not need to rely on inciting panic, fear, and anxiety; instead, it can transpire through co-construction, collaboration, and encouragement, as well as a clear vision and plan.

Racism and social inequalities can appear in the official accounts of an epidemic, especially when government officials otherize the responsibilities of contracting and spreading a virus to social minorities. For instance, the COVID-19 pandemic widened India's social, economic, and religious divides. Prime Minister Narendra Modi suppressed, harmed, and marginalized Muslims and migrant workers through different linguistic means, including "silence, presuppositions, accommodations, othering, dog-whistling, and povertyism" (Nagar, 2023, p. 321). In the Delta Amacuro of Venezuela, racism was a crucial factor that placed indigenous people at risk during the cholera epidemic from 1992 to 1993. Briggs and Mantini-Briggs' (2003) ethnographic studies show that the Warao ethnic group became an official scapegoat for cholera outbreaks. Public health and government officials attributed the epidemic cause to the Warao people's nomadic behavior and food customs of eating river crabs, which became entry points for connecting the epidemic to indigenous culture. The officials racialized the epidemic by sprinkling their epidemic accounts with Warao words (e.g., Noara, the annual celebration of the magical liturgical festival), which created the illusion that the officials understood what the Warao people thought, felt, and acted; scatological details, which generated an image of hygienic ignorance and resistance; and poetic parallelism in describing the movement of the Warao people, which evoked a sense of never-ending and careless migration.

Thus far, this literature review has shown the importance of metaphor and narrative in official accounts of an epidemic or pandemic, but government officials do not work alone in disseminating crisis information. Instead, they cooperate with media professionals to create biomediatization networks in which biomedical information becomes central to citizens' social lives. To illustrate the process of successful biomediatization, Briggs and Hallin (2016) analyzed H1N1 crisis communication in the United States in 2009. At that time, politicians and critics were generally sidelined while health and media professionals were well synchronized in their registers and discourses about H1N1. The biomediatization involved incorporating media logic into public health (e.g., practicing principles of emergency risk communication) and incorporating biomedicine into journalism (e.g., reading the US Centers for Disease Control and Prevention's Morbidity and Mortality Weekly Report). The collaboration between health officials and media professionals amplified public willingness to act according to official recommendations.

However, not all biomediatization is harmonious. At times, tensions lurk beneath the surface. A case in point is a Taiwanese journalist's blunt question during a COVID-19 press conference, as highlighted in my previous study (Lee, 2024b). After repeatedly questioning the official account of whether Taiwan's COVID-19 situation represented community spread, the journalist expressed frustration over an official's ambiguous response by restricting the ways in which the official could answer his question: 'If it is yes, just say yes. If it is no, just say no.' Moreover, government officials may change their language use to invite media attention, thereby forcing other officials to rectify their inaccurate data presentation. This was the case in the political manipulation of COVID-19 statistics by the health minister of the United Kingdom (Billig & Marinho, 2023). Additionally, when the pandemic presented many uncertainties that could not be accounted for by available evidence, health journalists and officials sometimes assumed divergent roles in handling speculation: speculative journalists, e.g., "What can you tell us about the virus. What makes it so dangerous?" versus fixed officials, e.g., "Well, in principle, you cannot even say that it is so dangerous at the moment. We don't know that much about the virus" (Blom et al., 2021). Thus, the relationships between health and media professionals are delicate and interdependent, consistently being negotiated according to the push and pull of information.

During an exclusive news interview, Dr. Yi-Chun Lo, deputy director-general and spokesperson for the Taiwan Centers for Disease Control (Taiwan CDC), who had regularly spoken at COVID-19 press conferences, recalled the challenge of keeping himself updated on the issues that were being discussed by news outlets so that he could be well prepared for journalists' questions at the daily press conferences (Formosa TV, 2022). Likewise, Dr. Allen Cheng, an epidemiologist in Australia, considered working with the media to be new and challenging when he stepped into the role of deputy chief health officer for the Victoria state government in 2020. Not only was his every word "scrutinized and dissected" by the media, but his previous position statements were quoted back to him for comments (Cheng, 2021, para. 6). The reflection of the officials on their time spent disseminating public health messages reinforces the importance of health officials and journalists co-creating a reciprocal network, instead of relying on a linear, top-down model of crisis information transmission.

This review of linguistic approaches to public health crisis discourse shows that metaphor and narrative have much to offer in understanding how government officials communicate and manage health crises. Racism and biomediatization are likewise garnering scholarly attention that is long overdue. To further elucidate the complexity of official health crisis communication and contribute to the existing discussion, throughout this book, I adopt the following measures. I explore how health officials use not just language but also gestures, eye gaze, and material artifacts to deliver health messages. I document the longitudinal challenges posed by COVID-19, ranging from devising initial responses to promoting approved actions that guided the public out of the crisis. I holistically study knowledge production, circulation, and reception. I further illustrate how the findings of discourse analytical research can have implications for the revision of existing guidelines on public health communication. Finally, I uncover an aspect of public health crisis discourse that has yet to receive sufficient attention but plays a decisive role in shaping official response and public perception: the practice of classification in press conferences.

What Kind of Classification?

Classification is about how a member of a professional group (e.g., archarologists or medical doctors) segments or orients toward the world (Bowker & Star, 1999; Goodwin, 2018) according to a system of categories or standards upheld by that group. Classification involves the processes of creating categorical types, delineating type relations, and sorting tokens into types. Bruner (1987) argued that in classification, "categories are established, instantiated, idealized, and related one to the other to form a system" (p. 12). Once types are created, tokens can be sorted into types or extracted from types if they do not fit. Classification thus entails a dialectical relationship between categorization and particularization. According to Billig (1985), categorization groups a single instance with other instances or in a general category, whereas particularization extracts a single instance from other instances or from a general category because the instance needs to be treated as a special case. Consider the presentation of COVID-19 statistics. Numbers can be tallied and linked to a category such as daily COVID-19 cases (categorization). The number of daily confirmed cases can also be extracted to present special categories such as local infection cases versus imported cases (particularization). Therefore, classification is inevitably rhetorical, and the rhetoric of comparison and contrast sits at the heart of classification.

Classification involves mental processes. In developmental psychology (Vygotsky, 1987), categories are considered conceptual knowledge created by human cultures to organize events and objects in the natural world. Categories thus represent the concepts of a particular social group and are made available to others through language learning. Lantolf and Poehner (2014) offered the following example to illustrate the relationship between the conceptual category and the natural world. The term "flower" is a superordinate category encompassing discrete entities such as roses, daisies, and tulips. Depending on the purpose of our communication, at times roses, daisies, and tulips are treated as discrete entities, and at other times they are treated as instantiations of the category of flower. Categories afford individuals greater flexibility in how they perceive and operate in the natural world. That is, one may adopt or abandon categories depending on the intentions of their interactions. Thus, our perception of the world is mediated by cultural concepts. For instance, throughout the COVID-19 pandemic, public health officials introduced SARS-CoV-2 variant classifications—WHO labels (e.g., Alpha, Beta, Gamma, and Delta) and Pango lineage (e.g., BA.2.86, XBB.1.9.1, and B.1.617.2)—to monitor the variants' impact on vaccines, therapeutics, and diagnostics (US Centers for Disease Control and Prevention, 2023) as well as help the public make sense of the continuously evolving situation of the pandemic.

In the same vein, Goodwin's (2018) multimodal research illustrates the transformation of sensory experience into categorical types and the socialization of individuals into competent actors who can operate with the inherited classification systems in the professional communities of archaeology, geology, and chemistry. In his research on professional vision, Goodwin meticulously uncovered how archaeologists adopted the Munsell chart to classify a patch of dirt and create a phenomenal object in their record. By doing so, the archaeologists transformed nature into culture.

If sensory experience can be shaped by sociocultural categories in communities, it can also be manipulated by individuals to achieve particular gains. In the research literature on COVID-19 discourse, two examples stand out as illustrative of this phenomenon. Billig (2021) showed that during the COVID-19 pandemic, politicians in the United Kingdom manipulated the use of round numbers for setting up goals such as the testing rate and precise numbers for achieving the goals. As such, quantitative categories such as round and precise numbers communicate qualitative categories such as good governance or bad governance. Similarly, Jones (2021c) presented an example of how the UK government failed to effectively communicate its message about COVID-19 through color-coded classification. The example Jones offered is the COVID-19 alert system, which consists of five levels ranging from Level 1 in green, which indicates no COVID-19 in the community, to Level 5 in red, which signals overwhelming risk to national health systems. The system shares its color-coded scheme with the terror alert system. However, the COVID-19 alert system does not provide specific details about the alert level, nor does it offer clear guidance on what actions people should take. As a result, it did not take long for the system to disappear from public discourse. Nevertheless, the COVID-19 alert system was used by the government as a performative tool for touting its competence in managing the crisis.

To uncover the functions of and rationale for classification, it is imperative to analyze the use of classification in social interaction. Membership categorization analysis (MCA) offers some useful concepts related to categorization. As a social interaction approach to categories, MCA explores people's "practices in describing the world, and displaying their understanding of the world and of the commonsense routine workings of society" (Fitzgerald et al., 2009, p. 47). While my focus in this book is on the introduction of categories that are novel to the public rather than commonsense reasoning, some key concepts in MCA discussed by Stokoe (2012) may be useful for understanding categorical reasoning and social actions at the COVID-19 press conferences I subsequently analyze. For example, categories can be organized hierarchically—for example, an imported case, a case of community infection, and a case of community spread, each of which indicates a different level of risk in the community. Categories can also be displayed in relational pairs, as when a journalist approached Taiwanese health officials, saying, 'I would like to ask if her symptoms appear to be mild or severe.' Moreover, categories are bounded by activities. This was the case when a Taiwanese official defined community spread as 'a risk of infection just by walking in the community.' Categories also have predicates or characteristics. Consider the example of a Taiwanese journalist who quoted other individuals to challenge health officials' introduction of a new numerical category related to the revised COVID-19 statistics: 'The retrospective adjustment looked like cooking the books.' These features suggest that categories oftentimes carry different "resonances and inferences" (Stokoe, 2012, p. 291) that can be uncovered by examining how individuals produce, invoke, orient to, receive, or resist categorical works.

Yet not all categories are based on commonsense knowledge and routine reasoning. Nor is classification only about the identities of members in a social group. Studies in science, technology, and medicine offer alternative views related to the production and emergence of novel classifications that help maintain social and moral order. Drawing on cases of diagnostic categories and statistics, Bowker and Star (1999) argued that classification is the temporal-spatial segmentation of the world through which knowledge and bureaucracy are produced. They proposed the notions of boundary objects and boundary infrastructures to highlight the dynamism of classification when classification systems are adopted by different social groups to encourage cooperation without consensus. Boundary objects are objects for cooperation. These objects maintain consistent identities but are loosely structured and adaptable to different communities of practice. Boundary infrastructures represent an expansion of boundary objects. They are larger infrastructures of classification that are institutionalized and embedded within the built environment. Classifying schemes that are used by health officials to determine pandemic situations and generate pandemic statistics are boundary objects and infrastructures *par excellence*. They are institutionalized categorical work that needs to be made adaptable to different communities of practice in order to mobilize public cooperation in perilous times.

Star and Bowker (1998) also argued that central to classification is the challenge of balancing vernacular terms with the formal structure of a classifying system. The example they provided is the diagnostic categories in the International Classification of Diseases. The development of the classification illustrates the conundrum of creating an unwieldy list to capture a range of only slightly different vernacular terms used by health practitioners worldwide and the necessity of creating a much shorter key for practitioners to use when filling out forms. In other words, classification inevitably involves embedding vernacular classifications in formal structures and vice versa. Indeed, such an embedding challenge also appeared at COVID-19 press conferences in Taiwan (Lee, 2024b). Consider this statement made at a COVID-19 press conference in Taiwan: 'Then there are also infections outside hospitals. They are called out-of-hospital infections. But this is called a community infection.' In this example, an epidemiologist strove to help the public understand the difference between community spread and community infection from a biomedical perspective. To do so, the epidemiologist continuously oscillated between folk classification (e.g., 'infections outside hospitals') and formal official classification (e.g., 'community infection').

Building on ideas about classification in anthropology, psychology, and sociology, this interdisciplinary book explores multimodal classification, which involves using language, narrative, numbers, gestures, eye gaze, and graphical representation to make invisible viruses and their transmission visible. I consider classification a multifaceted practice, not just in the mind but also in the social world, that is used to shape perception, cultivate competence, socialize membership, and foster cooperation across social groups. An important aim of the book is to pinpoint what multimodal features work or do not work in the process of making official classifications accessible to the public. To achieve this aim, throughout the book, I seek to answer the following questions:

1 What categories or standards constitute classification? What relationships exist among the categories and standards?
2 If categorization and particularization are assumed to be central to classification, how do these processes render some categories related but others unrelated?
3 How do different individuals (e.g., officials, journalists, and public online commenters) orient to the classification?
4 What happens when there is a discrepancy between the official and lay uses of a classification?
5 To what extent can health officials maximize the use of classification to foster cooperation across social groups?

I draw on Taiwanese examples of COVID-19 classifications to answer these questions.

Why Taiwan?

Every nation experienced the COVID-19 pandemic differently. China was ground zero of the pandemic in early 2020 but later declared victory over the disease, as it implemented lockdowns and mass testing, and the number of cases fell. However, the Chinese government's zero-COVID-19 policy provoked controversy as the rest of the world moved to co-exist with the virus (Ramzy, 2022). The United States' response to the pandemic confounded the world because the country was believed to have the most advanced doctors and technology but ended up with high morbidity and mortality rates as the pandemic became disastrously politicized (Healy et al., 2020). The pandemic was also a political crisis in the United Kingdom, where some politicians manipulated quantitative data for political gain (Billig, 2021; Billig & Marinho, 2023), and government officials gradually lost public trust because they breached their own lockdown policies (Seargeant, 2023). Both the leaders of the United States and the United Kingdom used illness narratives to depict themselves as strong and divert attention from discussions about their failure to formulate coherent plans for containing the virus (Jones, 2021b).

In addition to engaging in a soul-searching discussion of leadership failures, it is equally important to look beyond English-speaking countries to search for new definitions of effective official communication. Research that focuses on other countries has provided more favorable evaluations of pandemic leaders' responses, such as German Chancellor Angela Merkel's use of a dialogic frame (Wodak, 2021).

This book continues this line of research by detailing Taiwanese officials' strategies for COVID-19 crisis communication. Taiwan is an intriguing place to study because during the COVID-19 pandemic, international leaders and media outlets praised Taiwan's containment measures and referred to the measures as "the Taiwan model" (Berlinger, 2020; Manch, 2020). Throughout 2020, Taiwan did not enact strict restrictions but nevertheless was able to keep the infection largely at bay. The minister of health in Taiwan, Shih-Chung Chen, indicated that the Taiwan model was grounded in four principles: rapid measures, early deployment, prudent actions, and transparency (Chen, 2021). The Taiwan model also undercuts the argument that autocratic countries outperformed democratic countries in tackling the pandemic (cf. Song, 2020; Zheng, 2021). Taiwanese President Ing-wen Tsai emphasized that Taiwan adopted quarantine, contact tracing, and social distancing rather than the lockdowns and widespread testing common in China (Discovery, 2021). That is, the Taiwan model relied on clear guidelines that classified who should be subject to quarantine, whose contacts needed to be traced, and what distance should be kept during public social interactions.

However, just as Taiwanese officials were promoting their successes in combating COVID-19 without relying on draconian measures, the first large local outbreak was taking place. In the middle of 2021, the Taiwan model faced a series of challenges. The first large community outbreak since the start of the pandemic caught the government and the public by surprise. The outbreak, coupled with a shortage of vaccine doses, provoked domestic criticism of and skepticism about the government's policies. Conspiratorial accounts multiplied online with the aim of influencing public opinion about COVID-19 vaccines. Rampant accusations were made by political parties against other parties they thought had spread "disinformation" about the vaccines. Taiwan learned to mitigate the impact of COVID-19 and return to normal life through "the new Taiwan model" (Executive Yuan, 2022), but the dispute about its vaccine procurement practices lingered because the topic became highly politicized, especially during the election for the mayor of Taipei, the capital city of Taiwan. This book captures these key issues along the pathway of transitioning from the original Taiwan model to the new Taiwan model. The pathway reflects Taiwan's quest for international recognition and the disastrous entanglement of politics and health crisis communication.

Figure 1.1 represents this pathway with my English notation. It is a screenshot of a graph presented at a press conference on October 15, 2022, the thousandth day after the establishment of the Central Epidemic Command Center (CECC) to combat the pandemic. The CECC commander used the graph to characterize Taiwan's COVID-19 experience in three phases: transmission blocking, immunity enhancement, and virus coexistence. Each phase was defined according to different pandemic circumstances, including whether the vaccines had been developed or had become available and what types of COVID-19 variants were being transmitted. The graph also compares outbreaks in Taiwan with those throughout the rest of the world. The comparison underscores Taiwan's successes in pandemic management even before the vaccines had been developed.

Taiwan is also noteworthy due to its geographic proximity to and economic ties with China. The pandemic emerged in the middle of a trade war between China and the United States. Taiwan was carefully navigating its economic ties with both nations since its integrated circuits industry relies on factories and customers in China as well as equipment provided by the United States. Caught in the tension between the existing and emerging global superpowers, Taiwan had to tiptoe the superpowers' competition in vaccine diplomacy when Taiwan encountered a spike in cases and vaccine shortages.

Furthermore, the pandemic started to unfold right after the presidential election in Taiwan, in January 2020, when the ideological polarization of Taiwanese society was at its peak (Ko & Hsu, 2020). Similar to previous elections in Taiwan, the January 2020 presidential election boiled down to an ideological choice between two major political parties: the Nationalist Party of China (i.e., Kuomintang [KMT], or the blue party) versus the Demographic Progressive Party (i.e., DPP, or the green party). The KMT emphasizes Taiwan's identity as the Republic of China (Taiwan's official name) and supports closer ties with China, whereas the DPP stresses a uniquely Taiwanese identity and independence, thereby aligning itself more closely with democratic nations such as Japan and the United States. However, in comparison to the previous elections, the 2020 presidential election took on heightened importance because it immediately followed the 2019–2020 Hong Kong protests against the Hong Kong government's attempt to introduce a bill to amend the Fugitive Offenders Ordinance in regard to extradition. This amendment would have allowed the Chinese government to arrest political dissidents in

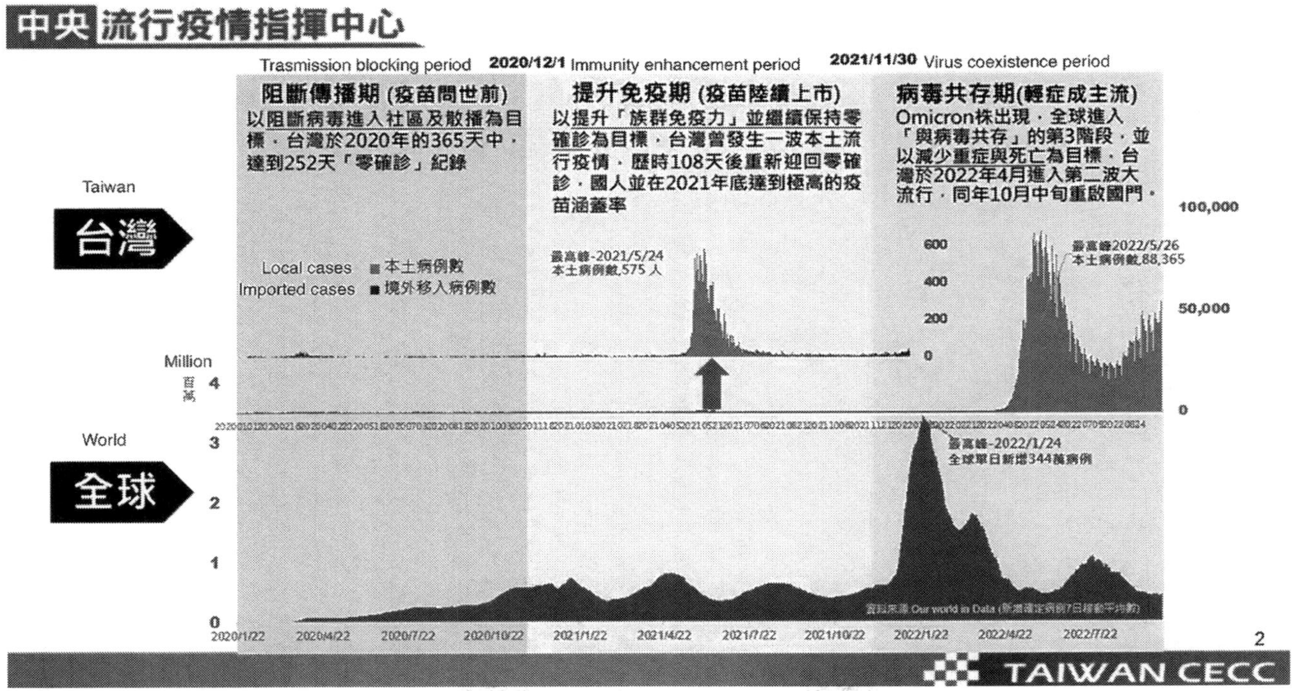

Figure 1.1 Taiwan's COVID-19 experience in three phases.

Source: Graph by the Taiwan Central Epidemic Command Center and used with permission from the Taiwan Centers for Disease Control. https://www.youtube.com/watch?v=v-mFymsa-Oc&t=863s

Hong Kong. The protests stoked fear in Taiwan as many Taiwanese were concerned that Taiwan would become like Hong Kong if they elected a person who was supportive of China (Ma, 2020). The international and domestic political circumstances worked in tandem to shape public stances, attitudes, and beliefs about the virus, vaccines, and health policies.

Taiwan's trauma from the 2003 SARS epidemic and the reforms enacted after the epidemic also made the book's focus on Taiwan logical, particularly as many nations have taken stock of the COVID-19 experience and strive to avoid repeating their mistakes in managing a public health crisis (Emanuel et al., 2023; Prime Minister's Office Singapore, 2023). Taiwan learned a hard lesson from the 2003 SARS epidemic. At that time, Taiwan suffered the third-largest outbreak in the world due to failures on multiple fronts, including public health systems, medical personnel, and acts of civility, such as hoarding masks and defying self-quarantine requirements (Fan & Chen, 2007; Ku & Wang, 2004). The chaotic response to the epidemic and the catastrophic loss of life propelled reforms in response plans for health crises, medical professional ethics, and public reflexive discussion about "uncivil" actions (Ku & Wang, 2004).

In a documentary (Taiwan Centers for Disease Control, 2021) that reviewed Taiwan's success in combating COVID-19 in 2020, a health official used the metaphor 磨劍十七年 'sharpening our swords for 17 years' to describe health officials' persistence and efforts in reforming the public health system and preparing for a public health emergency after the SARS epidemic. Another health official, who had been on the front lines of both the SARS epidemic and the COVID-19 pandemic commented in the documentary that 'public health is indeed an accumulation of experiences. Every twist and turn, we learn certain lessons and we fix it.' Just as health officials considered the lessons learned during SARS critical to their management of the COVID-19 pandemic, so too did health journalists draw on the SARS experience to help the public make sense of COVID-19. For example, when COVID-19 was ravaging China, Taiwanese news media recontextualized video footage of the SARS outbreak in order to remind the public of the importance of civic solidarity and moral responsibility (Lo & Hsieh, 2020). At early COVID-19 press conferences in Taiwan, it was not uncommon to observe journalists referencing their experience or knowledge of the 2003 SARS epidemic to seek official clarification on SARS-CoV-2, COVID-19 symptoms, and the latest policies.

Given the traumatic experience of the SARS epidemic, when confronted with the emergence of COVID-19 in 2020, the Taiwanese government acted quickly by adopting a centralized approach to avoid potential bureaucratic barriers to cooperation across governmental institutions. Central to this approach was the establishment of the Central Epidemic Command Center (CECC) to coordinate responses and resources. From 2020 to 2023, the CECC held 960 regular press conferences during which the organization allowed ample time for journalists' questions. These conferences were live-streamed online and broadcast on television. This represented a new and critical way of disseminating public health information in the digital era. As the conferences gradually became part of citizens' routine, or biomediatized, to use Briggs and Hallin's (2016) term, the quality of official communication also improved. Placards were created and used by health officials to underscore key information and untangle complex concepts. Subtitles and sign-language interpretation were incorporated into the conferences. In other words, visualizing and simplifying public health information was key to Taiwanese officials' crisis communication (Wei et al., 2022). The officials considered these ways of information dissemination as indicative of their commitment to the principles of transparency and immediacy in public health crisis communication.

Despite the amount of international attention paid to Taiwan's stellar performance in keeping the virus offshore, few studies explicitly focus on the linguistic and multimodal features used by Taiwanese officials to disseminate public health messages. Among these, Tseng (2023) analyzed official short videos that broadcast dos and don'ts to the public in Taiwan. His analysis convincingly showed that Taiwanese health officials' use of directives was infused with the sort of warm affectivity that is highly valued in Taiwan's society. In my past research, I have used multimodal discourse analysis to uncover the enregisterment of mask-wearing as a sign of civic solidarity and moral responsibility (Lee, 2023); the construction and circulation of pandemic detective narratives to repair public trust (Lee, 2024a); and the (de)construction of crisis classification over time in building public consensus (Lee, 2024b). Given the numerous successes and challenges associated with Taiwan's COVID-19 experience, a book that systematically details the multimodal features of Taiwan's crisis communication strategies will do justice to its efforts in combating COVID-19.

Data Collection and Triangulation

While COVID-19 broke out in China in January 2020, I was conducting an ethnographic study of Australian students studying abroad in Taiwan. Although there had been no outbreak in the community, I witnessed changes in life patterns there, partly because the 2003 SARS epidemic still haunted many Taiwanese. Soon after the news of the first Taiwanese COVID-19 case broke, hand sanitizer dispensers began to appear at the entrances to school buildings in Taiwan. Inside the classroom, pandemic registers such as the name of the virus and disease were introduced and discussed. Mask-wearing became commonplace at school and in public spaces. Some commercial establishments immediately implemented a requirement that patrons measure their body temperature before entering the premises—a containment measure commonly adopted during the 2003 SARS epidemic (Yang, 2003). COVID-19 dominated television news and the front pages of newspapers. Pandemic fear loomed large in everyday life.

Amid this mounting uncertainty about the virus spread and the urgent need to present a unified response to the health crisis, health officials held routine press conferences to disseminate information about COVID-19. Every day, a press conference was held at two o'clock in the afternoon. In early 2020, officials occasionally had to hold three conferences in a single day to make emergent announcements or clarifications. In late 2020, conferences were held once a week because the number of confirmed cases, if any, was usually in the single digits. In the subsequent years, the frequency of the conferences changed according to the pandemic situation. The last COVID-19 conference was held on April 27, 2023, because beginning in May 2023, COVID-19 was reclassified as a Level 4 communicable disease, putting it in the same category as influenza.

I began collecting videos of the COVID-19 press conferences in Taiwan when the conferences were live-broadcast by TV news reporters and streamed on social media platforms such as YouTube. The primary data used in this book are from this video corpus of COVID-19 press conference recordings. A research assistant and I collected 785 video recordings from the Taiwan Centers for Disease Control's YouTube account (www.youtube.com/@taiwancdc/videos) that aired from 2020 to 2023, yielding approximately 631 hours of footage. We also collected the online comments posted during these conferences in order to analyze how the public received and responded to the public health messaging. On YouTube, two types of comments are possible. There are comments left beneath the video, which usually focus on the overall content or key topics of the video. There are also live-chat responses to a specific segment of the livestreaming. Given my interest in classification practices, I focused on live-chat responses, as these show the commenters' immediate response to specific sequences of the conferences. I analyzed the more generic comments beneath the video if the live-chat function on a video had been disabled, such as when the first confirmed case of COVID-19 was reported (Chapter 2). Overall, we collected 2,197,037 live-chat responses and 1,008 comments beneath the video.

I also sought to uncover the communicative ideologies and models that underpinned Taiwan's health crisis communication. To this end, I consulted materials that represent health officials' high degree of reflexivity about health crisis communication. These materials include five memoirs (Chen & Lee, 2022; Huang, 2020; Taiwan Centers for Disease Control, 2024a, 2024b; Taiwan Ministry of Health and Welfare, 2022) and four documentaries or exclusive interviews on YouTube (BaoDao radio, 2024; Discovery Channel Taiwan, 2021; Formosa TV Thumbs Up, 2022; Taiwan Centers for Disease Control, 2021). Some of these materials were published by health officials themselves, their affiliated institutions, or the media. Collectively, these publications present officials' firsthand accounts, reflections, stances, and beliefs about pandemic communication. Their reflexivity adds precision to my analysis of press conference recordings and online comments.

Furthermore, I collected official documents about public health crisis communication that offer some suggestions for language use in health crisis communication, including the US Centers for Disease Control and Prevention's checklist of basic tenets of emergency risk communication (Reynolds, 2007) and its *Field Epidemiology Manual* (Tumpey et al., 2019). My online search of health communication guidelines in Taiwan turned up a limited number of official documents about health crisis communication. The only two documents containing such information usually are brief or generic in their guidelines for language use. For example, the Taiwan Centers for Disease Control (2020) released a document about contingency planning for the impending pandemic on February 28, 2020. One section in the document is about risk communication and features four strategies. One of the strategies is to

> [S]trengthen communication with the media. Regularly issue press releases and hold press conferences to explain current epidemic situations and corresponding measures. In addition, track public opinion continuously and proactively respond or clarify when necessary to avoid any misunderstanding or panic among the general public, and to effectively preserve community capacities. (Taiwan Centers for Disease Control, 2020, p. 10)

The lack of language and multimodal discussion about health crisis communication motivated the writing of this book. Here, I systematically lay out features of communicative strategies used by health officials at the press conferences and, more importantly, offer concrete suggestions for updating Taiwan's health crisis communication guidelines.

Thus, this book embodies the disposition of applied linguistics research by attending to issues that are real-world-relevant, problem-oriented, and language-centered (Brumfit, 1995). The disposition is materialized in one of the methods I have used: to study the processes of knowledge production, circulation, and reception in a backward order. I began with knowledge reception in order to identify communicative issues that had frequently been discussed in the media or online. These issues often generated polarized viewpoints or anxious uncertainties because information was limited at the time. For instance, Chapter 5 focuses on the purchase of the Pfizer-BioNTech COVID-19 vaccine, which received continuous media attention from 2020 to 2023 because many individuals held different views about the government's policies and practices. Chapter 4 analyzes the practices of 校正回歸 'retrospective adjustment' in presenting revised COVID-19 statistics, which garnered the largest online audience of any of the commander's utterances during the pandemic (Daileyview, 2022).

Having identified the issues that required investigation, I then sought to understand how knowledge circulation perpetuates or alleviates controversy and uncertainty. I searched for press conference recordings and news reports that involved various degrees of recontextualization. The search involved analyzing press-conference recordings across temporal scales (e.g., days, months, and even years) and digital news reports, such as online news articles and news videos uploaded to YouTube. Retracing knowledge circulation enabled me to understand what issues were left out and how some topics became distorted.

Finally, I zoomed in to study the production of knowledge in specific conference sequences. I attended to the ways in which health officials made claims to knowledge, health journalists sought to solicit and challenge official accounts, and both parties negotiated understanding in the push and pull of information exchanges.

To present a fuller picture of the life span of a classification, in each chapter, I triangulate my multimodal interaction analysis of press conferences with the thematic coding of live-chat responses and content analysis of public health communication materials. In analyzing the press conferences, I uncover the coordination of verbal and nonverbal channels by health officials and journalists. There are a variety of ways to study multimodal discourse (e.g., Mondada, 2016; Norris, 2019; van Leeuwen, 2005), but at the heart of all these approaches is the drive to understand meaning-making through the assemblage of multiple semiotic resources, not just language alone. Similarly, the analysis presented in the book emphasizes the semiotic configuration of multiple communicative resources used by health and media professionals as they strove to make sense of the relationship between official and lay classifications.

I transcribed various selected sequences of the conferences according to an adapted version of Du Bois et al.'s (1993) discourse transcription system. After transcribing the sequences, I analyzed each transcript and rewatched the footage with a focus on linguistic and multimodal features. By "linguistic features," I mean the linguistic elements and discursive patterns that are central to classifications such as metadiscourse, question formats, and stance-taking. By "multimodality," I mean speakers' hand shape, orientation, and motion (Kendo, 2004; McNeill, 2005; Streeck, 2009), as well as eye gaze and the speakers' use of material artifacts (Goodwin, 2018). Throughout the book, the transcribed sequences present each utterance in Chinese characters alongside its English translation. To enhance the readability of the translation, I changed the English syntax or inserted additional English words in parentheses whenever necessary. I placed photos of multimodal features beneath the utterances that co-occurred with the use of the features. The specific parts of an utterance that overlap with the multimodal features are underlined. The order of the photos is from left to right, and gesture or eye movement is labeled with dotted red arrows.

Regarding public responses, I extracted the comments beneath press conference videos on YouTube and the online live-chat responses that were posted in reaction to each specific sequence of the press conferences. Subsequently, I removed the same and repetitive responses by the commenters such as spammers, and categorized the remaining responses according to themes. In my analysis, I present examples of online responses to show how a conference sequence was received. To preclude any retracing of usernames online, I present only the English translation of the comments. It is important to note that my presentation of online comments is not exhaustive because I am unable to include examples of all identified themes. Instead, I focus on comments that are directly relevant to classifications, conspiracies, and metapragmatics (Caffi, 1994; Verschueren, 2022), i.e., reflexive interpretations or judgements of appropriateness on communicative behavior. These comments show the commenters' reception of official classifications and perceptions of officials' and journalists' communication styles.

Regarding the public health communication materials, I concentrate on the specific communicative principles presented in these materials by comparing and contrasting the principles with the findings of my multimodal and thematic analyses. I also identify gaps in the principles—places where no communicative strategies are offered to address communicative challenges that may arise at press conferences. In such cases, I make suggestions to fill in the gaps. By triangulating these three types of data and analyses—i.e., multimodal conferences, online responses, and communicative principles—I am able to uncover the strengths and weaknesses of existing ideologies about and resources for health crisis communication.

Outline of the Book

The book is structured according to different aspects of classification used in health crisis communication. Because each chapter serves as its own case study, the chapters may productively be read out of order. However, some readers may find it lends clarity to the argument if they begin with the production of classification through the interaction between health officials and journalists (Chapter 2), proceed to the combination of classification with other genres including narrative (Chapter 3)and numbers talk (Chapter 4), and finally read about the circulation of classification (Chapter 5). The key content in each chapter is summarized below to help readers decide their reading preferences.

In Chapter 2, I analyze the interaction between health journalists and public health officials at press conferences in Taiwan and the public reception of this interaction. Focusing on the first case, the first community-acquired infection, and the first death during the first wave of the COVID-19 outbreak in 2020, I identify discourses that capture the medical conditions of individuals with COVID-19 and the crisis status of the community. To account for the biomediatization of these discourses, I propose a framework characterizing discursive practices between journalists and officials in their negotiation of classifications: (1) disjunctive questions erase categorical entanglements and enhance newsworthiness; (2) metadiscursive framing inscribes journalistic initiative into interaction; (3) biocommunicable relationships are recalibrated to index officials' authority and credibility; and (4) multimodal signs synchronize with speech to objectify biomedical phenomena and reify subject positions. Although they collide at times, these discursive processes construct a network of biomedical objects and subjects for alerting and reassuring the public. The push and pull of COVID-19 classification between journalists and officials organizes the categorical configuration of and response to the crisis.

Chapter 3 explores the interface of classification and narration in communicating COVID-19 restrictions on human mobility. The interface embodies Bruner's (1987) two modes of thought: paradigmatic and narrative. Paradigmatic thinking is concerned with objective, universal truth, whereas narrative reasoning pursues lifelikeness. The modes are dialectically intertwined to help individuals make sense of the world. Drawing on this dialectic, I study the controversy surrounding the Taiwanese government's revised restrictions on mobility that allowed minor children of Chinese and Taiwanese couples to enter Taiwan during the initial outbreak of the COVID-19 pandemic. I analyze how a government official attempted to use classification and narration to convince the public of the change but instead sparked criticism and confusion by unwittingly portraying the children as ungrateful outsiders who benefited from Taiwan's social welfare system but did not identify with Taiwan. In this sense, the classification was devoid of verification and congruence. Adopting a narrative classification framework to analyze the episode, in this chapter I uncover the complexities of engendering pandemic identities that mediate the public reception of health crisis restrictions.

Chapter 4 focuses on numbers from a qualitative perspective. During the COVID-19 outbreak, there was criticism of official measures and policies based on incomplete or inaccurate data. What happened when public health officials realized the statistics were wrong? How, if at all, did they explain the incompleteness and inaccuracy to the public, and were they successful? In this chapter, I analyze a Taiwanese public health official's multimodal classification of daily case numbers that were incomplete and needed to be revised. The official classified the revised numbers as a case of retrospective adjustment, which provoked both public support and criticism. To quell public criticism, the official then contextualized the classification using narratives, graphs, gestures, and metadiscourse. The contextualization aggregated and disaggregated numbers to form different numerical patterns and categorical relations, which in turn enabled the official and his public health colleagues to communicate their control of the outbreak progression and the fleetingness of time. These qualities of numerical classification suggest that numbers are not merely decontextualized variables or representative of cold logicality. Instead, through classification, numbers are infused with particular qualitative meanings and set in relation to past, present, and hypothetical time. However, it is also through these meanings that numbers become open to reinterpretation and even contestation.

Chapter 5 approaches issues of vaccine branding and false information through the lens of classification. I propose the concept of *classification in mobility* to elucidate the processes of disseminating classifications during a health emergency. There are two aspects of mobility I consider: production and circulation. In production, I focus on the metadiscursive practices of making some categories mobile and others immobile. In circulation, I trace the act of recontextualization, which involves extracting a text about classification from its discursive context and inserting the text into a new context. To illustrate this mobility, I draw on an episode about the purchase of the Pfizer–BioNTech COVID-19 vaccine from BioNTech in Germany and Shanghai Fosun Pharma in China. Specifically, I show how over the course of three years, government officials first wrestled with the classification of the vaccine as German, then confronted the conundrum of naming the vaccine in Chinese or German, and finally impeded the circulation of the vaccine's Chinese trade name in simplified characters—i.e., 复必泰 'Fubitai'—a name which is associated with Chinese manufacturing. Along the way, conspiratorial accounts about the government's plan for vaccine procurement multiplied online. Expressions such as "disinformation" and "conspiracy theories" were used by political parties and online commenters to politicize public health communication. I account for the processes based on three semiotic types: symbolic authority, indexical multiplicity, and iconic veracity. Symbolic authority emerged in the officials' use of institutional power and industry norms to quell speculation. Indexical multiplicity appeared primarily when journalists solicited and challenged officials' accounts. Iconic veracity perpetuated disputes over whose account better represented the reality of the BioNTech vaccine purchase. These semiotic types constellated to create unique circuits of vaccine classification, and studying them offers fresh insights into contentious issues about vaccine branding and false information in Taiwan.

Chapter 6, the last chapter of the book, summarizes the key findings of my research and discusses their implications for crisis communication in public health. I synthesize the analytical chapters by distilling areas of commonality and variation. The synthesis is structured according to the production, circulation, and reception of pandemic classifications. Drawing on my findings and building on existing principles of public health communication, I offer five suggestions for public health practitioners. In doing so, I depart from the academic prose in other sections of the book, speaking directly to practitioners in a way that is more likely to be useful for future public health communication.

Note

1 Single quotation marks, if not used within a quote, indicate English translation of Chinese.

References

Adams, P. (2020, April 3). *The PM's metaphorical view of Covid-19*. newsroom. https://newsroom.co.nz/2020/06/02/the-pms-metaphorical-view-of-covid-19/

BaoDao radio. (2024, April 23). 【寶島全世界】回憶*covid-19*大流行，王必勝：防疫工作，有一半在處理政治攻防！來賓：王必勝　衛服部政務次長 | 鄭弘儀主持 *2024/04/23* [Formosa Around the World] Victor Wang reflecting on the COVID-19 pandemic: 'Half of epidemic prevention work was about dealing with political infighting!' Guest: Victor Wang, deputy minister of the ministry of health and welfare | Hosted by Jeng, Hung-Yi, 2024/04/23] [Video]. YouTube. www.youtube.com/watch?v=T3VAjaHb49Q

Berlinger, J. (2020, October 30). *Taiwan just went 200 days without a locally transmitted Covid-19 case. Here's how they did it.* CNN. https://edition.cnn.com/2020/10/29/asia/taiwan-covid-19-intl-hnk/index.html

Billig, M. (1985). Prejudice, categorization and particularization: From a perceptual to a rhetorical approach. *European Journal of Social Psychology*, *15*(1), 79–103. https://doi.org/10.1002/ejsp.2420150107

Billig, M. (2021). Rhetorical uses of precise numbers and semi-magical round numbers in political discourse about COVID-19: Examples from the government of the United Kingdom. *Discourse & society*, *32*(5), 542–558. https://doi.org/10.1177/09579265211013115

Billig, M., & Marinho, C. (2023). Preventing the political manipulation of Covid-19 statistics: The importance of going beyond diplomatic language. *Language in Society*, *52*(5), 733–755. https://doi.org/10.1017/S0047404522000367

Black, S. P. (2019). *Speech and song at the margins of global health: Zulu tradition, HIV stigma, and AIDS activism in South Africa*. Rutgers University Press.

Blom, J. N., Rønlev, R., Hansen, K. R., & Ljungdalh, A. K. (2021). The potentials and pitfalls of interactional speculations by journalists and experts in the media: The case of Covid-19. *Journalism Studies*, *22*(9), 1142–1160. https://doi.org/10.1080/1461670X.2021.1925950

Bowker, G. C., & Star, S. L. (1999). *Sorting things out: Classification and its consequences.* MIT Press.

Briggs, C. L. (2024). *Incommunicable: Toward communicative justice in health and medicine*. Duke University Press. https://doi.org/10.1215/9781478059240

Briggs, C. L., & Hallin, D. C. (2016). *Making health public: How news coverage is remaking media, medicine, and contemporary life.* Routledge. https://doi.org/10.4324/9781315658049

Briggs, C. L., & Mantini-Briggs, C. (2003). *Stories in the time of Cholera: Racial profiling during a medical nightmare.* University of California Press. https://doi.org/10.1525/9780520938526

Brumfit, C. J. (1995). Teacher professionalism and research. In G. Cook & B. Seidlhofer (Eds.), *Principle and practice in applied linguistics* (pp. 27–42). Oxford University Press.

Bruner, J. (1987). *Actual minds, possible worlds.* Harvard University Press.

Buruma, I. (2020, March 28). Virus as metaphor. *The New York Times.* www.nytimes.com/2020/03/28/opinion/coronavirus-racism-covid.html

Caffi, C. (1994). Metapragmatics. In R. E. Asher (Ed.), *Encyclopedia of language and linguistics* (2nd ed., pp. 2461–2466). Pergamon. https://doi.org/10.1016/B0-08-044854-2/00317-5

Charteris-Black, J. (2021). *Metaphors of coronavirus: Invisible enemy or zombie apocalypse?*. Springer Nature. https://doi.org/10.1007/978-3-030-85106-4

Chen, S.-C. (2021). Taiwan's experience in fighting COVID-19. *Nature Immunology*, *22*, 393–394. https://doi.org/10.1038/s41590-021-00908-2

Chen, S.-C., & Lee, C.-Q. (2022). 溫暖的魄力：陳時中的從醫初心 [Warm determination: Chen Shih-Chung's initial aspiration of becoming a doctor]. Commonwealth Publishing Group.

Cheng, A. (2021, September 6). *My year as Victoria's deputy chief health officer: On the pandemic, press conferences and our COVID future.* The Conversation. https://theconversation.com/my-year-as-victorias-deputy-chief-health-officer-on-the-pandemic-press-conferences-and-our-covid-future-166164

Chiang, W.-Y., & Duann, R.-F. (2007). Conceptual metaphors for SARS: "war" between whom? *Discourse & Society*, *18*(5), 579–602. https://doi.org/10.1177/0957926507079631

Clayman, S. E. (2002). Tribune of the people: Maintaining the legitimacy of aggressive journalism. *Media, Culture & Society*, *24*(2), 197–216. https://doi.org/10.1177/016344370202400203

Collins, L. C., & Koller, V. (2023). *Viral language: Analysing the Covid-19 pandemic in public discourse*. Routledge. https://doi.org/10.4324/9781003163459

Dailyview. (2022, July 24). 陳時中十大防疫金句連發！網友討論度最高的是這句話…… *[Top 10 iconic quotes of pandemic prevention by Shih-Chung Chen! This one sparked most online discussion……]*. https://dailyview.tw/daily/3411

Discovery Channel Taiwan. (2021, January 26). *BEATING COVID-19* 台灣戰疫全紀錄 完整版 上集 [BEATING COVID-19 A complete record of Taiwan's battle against the pandemic, full version, part 1.] [Video]. YouTube. www.youtube.com/watch?v=xJGoZhL7TOo

Du Bois, J. W., Schuetze-Coburn, S., Cumming, S., & Paolino, D. (1993). Outline of discourse transcription. In J. A. Edwards & M. D. Lampert (Eds.), *Talking data: Transcription and coding in discourse research* (pp. 45–89). Lawrence Erlbaum Associates. https://doi.org/10.4324/9781315807928

Emanuel, E. J., Borio, L., Bright., R., Osterholm, M. T., Jim, J., & Michaels, D. (2023, May 11). We worked on the US pandemic response. Here are 13 takeaways for the next health emergency. *The New York Times*. www.nytimes.com/2023/05/11/opinion/covid-pandemic-lessons.html

Executive Yuan. (2022). *Government pushes 'new Taiwan model' of zero severe COVID cases and effective management of mild cases*. https://english.ey.gov.tw/Page/61BF20C3E89B856/30b342f1-1261-408c-b915-a61a9af78e29

Fan, Y., & Chen, M.-C. (2007). The weakness of a post-authoritarian democratic society: Reflections upon Taiwan's societal crisis during the SARS outbreak. In D. Davis & H. F. Siu (Eds.), *SARS: Reception and interpretation in three Chinese cities* (pp. 147–64). Routledge.

Fitzgerald, R., Housley, W., & Butler, C. W. (2009). Omnirelevance and interactional context. *Australian Journal of Communication*, *36*(3), 45–64.

Formosa TV Thumbs Up. (2022, March 28). *【新聞觀測站】堅守疫戰前線！疾管署副署長羅一鈞獨家專訪 2022.3.26* [News observatory. Holding the frontline in the fight against the pandemic! Exclusive interview with the CDC deputy director Yi-Chun Lo] [Video]. YouTube. www.youtube.com/watch?v=B9aBk0QsMRk&t=39s

Goodwin, C. (2018). *Co-Operative action*. Cambridge University Press. https://doi.org/10.1017/9781139016735

Hafner, C. A., & Sun, T. (2021). The 'team of 5 million': The joint construction of leadership discourse during the Covid-19 pandemic in New Zealand. *Discourse, Context & Media*, *43*, 100523. https://doi.org/10.1016/j.dcm.2021.100523

Hanne, M. (2022). How we escape capture by the "war" metaphor for Covid-19. *Metaphor and Symbol*, *37*(2), 88–100. https://doi.org/10.1080/10926488.2021.1935261

Healy, J., Robertson, C., & Tavernise, S. (2020, March 1). How coronavirus is already being viewed through a partisan lens. *The New York Times*. www.nytimes.com/2020/03/01/us/coronavirus-us-politics.html

Higgins, C., & Norton, B. (2010). *Language and HIV/AIDS*. Multilingual Matters.

Huang, G.-Q. (2020). 戰疫：鐵人部長陳時中與台灣抗疫英雄們 *[Pandemic battle: Shih-Chung Chen, the iron minister, and Taiwan's heroes of the fight]*. Commonwealth Publishing Group.

Jenkins, S. (2020, March 7). Why I'm taking the coronavirus hype with a pinch of salt. *The Guardian*. www.theguardian.com/commentisfree/2020/mar/06/coronavirus-hype-crisis-predictions-sars-swine-flu-panics

Jones, R. H. (Ed.). (2021a). *Viral discourse*. Cambridge University Press. https://doi.org/10.1017/9781108986465

Jones, R. H. (2021b). The wounded leader: The illness narratives of Boris Johnson and Donald Trump. *Discourse, Context & Media*, *41*, 100499. https://doi.org/10.1016/j.dcm.2021.100499

Jones, R. H. (2021c). Order out of chaos: Coronavirus communication and the construction of competence. In R. H. Jones (Ed.) *Viral discourse* (pp. 69–78). Cambridge University Press. https://doi.org/10.1016/j.dcm.2021.100499

Kendon, A. (2004). *Gesture: Visible action as utterance*. Cambridge University Press. https://doi.org/10.1017/CBO9780511807572

Ko, H.-H., & Hsu, C.-Y. (2020, January 8). 選舉語言的祕密：解析韓國瑜、蔡英文圈粉術 *[Secrets of election language: Analyzing Kuo-Yu Han and Ing-Wen Tsai's strategies for winning support]*. The Reporter. www.twreporter.org/a/2020-election-politician-art-of-speech

Ku, A. S., & Wang, H.-L. (2004). The making and unmaking of civic solidarity: Comparing the coping responses of civil societies in Hong Kong and Taiwan during the SARS crises. *Asian Perspective*, *28*(1), 121–147. https://dx.doi.org/10.1353/apr.2004.0036

Lantolf, J. P., & Poehner, M. E. (2014). *Sociocultural theory and the pedagogical imperative in L2 education: Vygotskian praxis and the research/practice divide*. Routledge. https://doi.org/10.4324/9780203813850

Lee, S.-H. (2023). Enregistering mask-wearing in the time of a public health crisis. *Language in Society*, *52*(3), 485–509. https://doi.org/10.1017/S0047404522000033

Lee, S.-H. (2024a). How pandemic detective narratives potentiate and debilitate trust. *Text & Talk*, *44*(6), 809–841. https://doi.org/10.1515/text-2022-0080

Lee, S.-H. (2024b). Crisis classifications in mobility: Reporting the first COVID death in Taiwan. *Discourse Studies*, *26*(2), 242–261. https://doi.org/10.1177/14614456231219741

Liu, R.-Y. (2024). Constituting institutional identity in political discourse: The use of the first-person plural pronoun in China's press conferences. *Language in Society*, *53*(3), 421–444. https://doi.org/10.1017/S0047404523000386

Lo, M.-C. M., & Hsieh, H.-Y. (2020). The "Societalization" of pandemic unpreparedness: Lessons from Taiwan's COVID response. *American Journal of Cultural Sociology*, *8*, 384–404. https://doi.org/10.1057/s41290-020-00113-y

Ma, Y. (2020, November 26). 《反抗的共同體》：反送中營造出「亡國感」，幫助蔡英文破紀錄*817*萬票連任 *[Community of resistance: How anti-txtradition movement created "sense of national crisis," helping Ing-Wen Tsai secure record-breaking 8.17 million votes for re-election]*. The News Lens. www.thenewslens.com/article/143468

Manch, T. (2020, March 15). *Coronavirus: New Zealand likely to follow Taiwan in advising cancellation of crowded gatherings*. Stuff. www.stuff.co.nz/national/health/coronavirus/120294477/coronavirus-new-zealand-likely-to-follow-taiwan-in-advising-cancellation-of-crowded-gatherings.html

McNeill, D. (2005). *Gesture and thought.* University of Chicago Press.

Mondada, L. (2016). Challenges of multimodality: Language and the body in social interaction. *Journal of sociolinguistics, 20*(3), 336–366. https://doi.org/10.1111/josl.1_12177

Nagar, I. (2023). The language of suppression: Muslims, migrant workers, and India's response to COVID-19. *Language in Society, 52*(2), 321–344. https://doi.org/10.1017/S0047404521000816

Norris, S. (2019). *Systematically working with multimodal data: Research methods in multimodal discourse analysis.* John Wiley & Sons.

Olza, I., Koller, V., Ibarretxe-Antuñano, I., Pérez-Sobrino, P., & Semino, E. (2021). The # reframe Covid initiative: From Twitter to society via metaphor. *Metaphor and the Social World, 11*(1), 98–120. https://doi.org/10.1075/msw.00013.olz

Paulus, D. (2020, May 22). *How politicians talk about coronavirus in Germany, where war metaphors are avoided.* The Conversation.https://theconversation.com/how-politicians-talk-about-coronavirus-in-germany-where-war-metaphors-are-avoided-137427

Prime Minister's Office Singapore. (2023, March 8). *White paper on Singapore's response to COVID-19: Preparing Singapore better for the next pandemic.* www.pmo.gov.sg/Newsroom/Release-on-White-Paper-on-Singapore-response-to-COVID-19

Ramzy, A. (2022, September 8). China's zero-Covid approach explained. *The New York Times.* www.nytimes.com/2022/09/08/world/asia/china-zero-covid-explainer.html

Reynolds, B. (2007). *Crisis and emergency risk communication: Pandemic influenza.* https://stacks.cdc.gov/view/cdc/7037

Seargeant, P. (2023). *Crisis leadership: Boris Johnson and political persuasion during the Covid pandemic.* Cambridge University Press. https://doi.org/10.1017/9781009321983

Song, L. (2020, March 15). Many Western governments ill-equipped to handle coronavirus. *Global Times.* www.globaltimes.cn/content/1182661.shtml

Sontag, S. (1978). *Illness as metaphor.* Farrar, Straus and Giroux.

Star, S. L., & Bowker, G. C. (1998). Introduction. *Library Trends, 47*(2), 185–189.

Stokoe, E. (2012). Moving forward with membership categorization analysis: Methods for systematic analysis. *Discourse Studies, 14*(3), 277–303. https://doi.org/10.1177/1461445612441534

Streeck, J. (2009). *Gesturecraft: The manu-facture of meaning.* John Benjamins. https://doi.org/10.1075/gs.2

Taiwan Centers for Disease Control. (2020). *Preparedness and contingency planning in response to COVID-19 epidemic.* www.cdc.gov.tw/File/Get/JFnBQLuyGNcuROKLUMjuhA

Taiwan Centers for Disease Control. (2021, January 14). | *TRusT* | *Documentary on one-year anniversary of Taiwan's fight against COVID-19* | *English version* [Video]. YouTube. www.youtube.com/watch?v=4Obtht6e_d0

Taiwan Centers for Disease Control. (2024a). 後疫情時代防疫政策白皮書 *[White paper on Taiwan's epidemic prevention policy in post-COVID-19 era].* Taiwan Centers for Disease Control.

Taiwan Centers for Disease Control. (2024b). 疫起走過 *COVID-19* 嚴重特殊傳染性肺炎大流行工作紀實 *[Navigating the pandemic together: Taiwan's response to the COVID-19].* Taiwan Centers for Disease Control.

Taiwan Ministry of Health and Welfare. (2022). 戰疫堡壘 *[Fortress against the pandemic].* Taiwan Ministry of Health and Welfare.

Tseng, M. Y. (2023). Rén qíng wèi ('flavour of human feelings') in the pragmeme of delivering Covid-19 directives. *Journal of Pragmatics*, *218*, 31–44. https://doi.org/10.1016/j.pragma.2023.09.018

Tumpey, A. J., Daigle, D., & Nowak, G. (2019). Communicating during an outbreak or public health investigation. In S. A. Rasmussen & R. A. Goodman (Eds.), *The CDC field epidemiology manual* (pp. 243–260). Oxford University Press. https://doi.org/10.1093/oso/9780190933692.001.0001

US Centers for Disease Control and Prevention. (2023, September 1). *SARS-CoV-2 variant classifications and definitions.* https://stacks.cdc.gov/view/cdc/133705/cdc_133705_DS1.pdf

van Leeuwen, T. (2005). *Introducing social semiotics: An introductory textbook.* Routledge.

Vásquez, C. (2021). Leading with stories: Andrew Cuomo, family narratives and authentic leadership. *Discourse, Context & Media*, *41*, 100507. https://doi.org/10.1016/j.dcm.2021.100507

Verschueren, J. (2022). Metapragmatics. In J. Verschueren & J.-O. Östman (Eds.), *Handbook of pragmatics: Manual* (2nd ed., pp. 948–953). John Benjamins. https://doi.org/10.1075/hop.m.met1

Vygotsky, L. S. (1987). *The collected works of L. S. Vygotsky. Volume 1: Problems of general psychology, including the volume thinking and speech.* R. W. Rieber & A. S. Carton (Eds.). Plenum. https://doi.org/10.1007/978-1-4613-1655-8

Wallace-Wells, D. (2023, January 4). 9 Pandemic narratives we're getting wrong. *The New York Times.* www.nytimes.com/2023/01/04/opinion/covid-pandemic-history.html?searchResultPosition=20

Wei, H.-N., Dai, Y.-S., Ko, H.-Y., & Tsao, K.-L. (2022). 運用新媒體進行 COVID-19疫情相關衛教及溝通 [Uusing new media for COVID-19-related health education and communication]. *Taiwan Epidemiology Bulletin*, *38*(24), 359–376.

Wodak, R. (2021). Crisis communication and crisis management during COVID-19. *Global Discourse*, *11*(3), 329–353. https://doi.org/10.1332/204378921X16100431230102

Yang, M.-Y. (2003, June 16). 今天你幾度？ *[What is your temperature today?].* BBC Chinese. http://news.bbc.co.uk/hi/chinese/china_news/newsid_2993000/29934802.stm

Zheng, W. (2021, May 6). Xi Jinping says China is 'invincible', regardless of challenges ahead. *South China Morning Post.* www.scmp.com/news/china/politics/article/3132383/xi-jinping-says-china-invincible-regardless-challenges-ahead

2 The Push and Pull of COVID-19 Classifications

This chapter focuses on the emergence and interpretation of health-crisis classifications at three critical moments during the first wave of COVID-19 outbreaks: the identification of the first case, the first community-acquired infection, and the first death. These classifications attract public spectacle as their categories are radiated out of press conferences to shape public behaviors and discourses. A deeper understanding of how such classifications emerge in the interaction between journalists and officials at press conferences has implications for effectively communicating and managing public health information when little is known about the encroaching threat, and much remains uncertain about the eventual trajectory of the crisis situation.

Prior scholarship has examined the entanglement of media and public health. In their landmark book about the metapragmatics of making health knowledge public, Briggs and Hallin (2016) presented health officials' characterization of interacting with journalists as "push" (disseminating official messages) vs. "pull" (responding to journalists' inquiries). This push and pull represents one of the many norms assumed by health officials when interpreting the production, circulation, and reception of health information, also known as *biocommunicability* (Briggs & Hallin, 2016). Other norms include who has the authority to produce health knowledge, whether affect can be embedded in public health communication, and what modes of communication should be adopted (e.g., creating press releases, holding press conferences, or producing health advertisements). Further complexifying biocommunicability is the reality that health information does not flow linearly from scientists to the general public. Instead, it is *biomediatized*. Biomediatization is a process of creating medical objects and subjects that have both biological and media components through collaborations among actors such as health and media professionals (Briggs & Mantini-Briggs, 2016). In this process, different individuals assume different biocommunicable roles. For instance, while health journalists are likely to be positioned as the transmitters of health information, health journalists may perceive themselves to be translators, fraud detectors, the eyes and ears of the public, or members of the health education team (Briggs, 2011). If journalists not only report but also engage in the process of

DOI: 10.4324/9781003545002-2

producing and circulating medical objects and subjects, how do they arrive at full, accurate, and firsthand information without being overly pushy or adversarial? To what extent can public health officials be forthcoming in responding to journalists' questions without provoking public panic?

To explore and theorize the intricacies of the interaction between journalists and officials, in this chapter, I draw on examples of question-and-answer sequences from COVID-19 press conferences. I illustrate how speech works in tandem with multimodal signs to produce, challenge, and circulate pandemic-related categories. My focus on three "first" times (i.e., first confirmed case, first community-acquired infection, and first death) demonstrates how health journalists and officials engage in these sequences when existing and emerging classifications are in discord and when both parties are under the immense pressure of accounting for pandemic detection, transmission, and death.

In what follows, I first propose a framework for interpreting classifications in the push and pull between officials and journalists. I then provide contextual information to help readers understand against what background the push and pull of COVID-19 classification emerges. Subsequently, I present my analysis to illustrate the push and pull of COVID-19 discourses as health officials and the press negotiate categorical boundaries and online commenters engage in the negotiation by sharing their interpretation of the interaction. Finally, I summarize key findings and extrapolate implications.

Push and Pull Between Officials and Journalists

Throughout the COVID-19 pandemic, press conferences were a critical means by which government officials provided updates, contained misinformation, reassured citizens, and announced health measures (Dau & Ellis, 2023). The conferences also provided a venue for journalists to hold officials accountable and for the public to directly participate in crisis communication, particularly in the age of live-streaming. Given these important functions, daily press conferences at some points during the pandemic became must-watch media events (Lu, 2020; Wei et al., 2022).

The typical format of a press conference was an official presentation followed by a question-and-answer session with journalists. Emerging studies on COVID-19 press conferences have uncovered linguistic and rhetorical features of such official presentations, which were intended to update pandemic statuses and mobilize community cooperation (e.g., Degani, 2022; Vásquez, 2021). However, the question-and-answer session has not received an equal amount of research attention. Without investigating the interactions during the question-and-answer period, scholars have only a partial understanding of pandemic press conferences. We do not know whether journalistic questioning in health crisis communication is as direct, assertive, and hostile as it is in political discourse (Clayman & Heritage, 2002). Do journalists "preformulate" (Jacobs, 1999, p. xii) certain categories—i.e., how the categories in official response are anticipated—to push for a particular response in the course of questioning? Why might certain interactional practices work to the advantage of officials as they evade confrontational questions that involve sensitive subjects, call into question their credibility, or expose inconsistencies (Bhatia, 2006)?

The question-and-answer session during a press conference is a power maneuver between officials and journalists. As part of this maneuver, control might be asserted by referencing authoritative sources (e.g., World Health Organization) or evoking identities (e.g., nationalities), thereby recreating biocommunicable cartographies (Briggs & Hallin, 2016) that show how biomedical information is constructed, circulated, and received at particular subjective positions. Ideally, the question-and-answer session renders public health crisis communication a two-way exchange between officials and communities rather than a one-way attempt at information transmission that assumes the public to be ignorant and the health officials to be authoritative (Hyland-Worrd et al., 2021). However, the exchanges during the question-and-answer period can also turn press conferences into contentious sites. For instance, US President Donald Trump accused a reporter of asking "a nasty question" and then refused to answer questions from any other reporters, instead abruptly ending his COVID-19 conference (Wilkie, 2020, para. 12). Donald Trump might be an exceptional case because attacking the media has been his hallmark since his first presidential campaign (Kalb, 2018), but consider an example from Taiwan's Central Epidemic Command Center, which had been commended for its openness and transparency in pandemic communication (Griffiths, 2020; Wang et al., 2020). At a daily COVID-19 press conference, the center's then-spokesperson, Dr. Chuang Jen-hsiang, said, 我為什麼要告訴你? 'Why do I have to tell you?' in response to a journalist's question regarding the number of countries in which administration of the AstraZeneca vaccine had been temporarily halted due to the side effect of unintentional blood clotting (T.-Y. Lee, 2021, para. 1). The spokesperson's response was heavily criticized by online viewers of the conference and politicians of the opposition party. As a result, the spokesperson apologized to the public in a subsequent press conference. These examples suggest that knowing how to strategically negotiate the question-and-answer session is as important as being able to present key messages during a press conference on a public health crisis.

A common way of conceptualizing question-and-answer interactions at a press conference is push and pull. Blom et al. (2021) investigated assertive and tentative speculations between journalists and health experts in Denmark during the initial outbreak of COVID-19. They proposed a model of the push-and-pull mechanism to explain that once a speculation has been lobbed, it can be either accelerated (push) or decelerated (pull). In the model, pushing is about asserting without reservations or expressing confidence, saying, for example, "It is not the case that the virus is in Denmark." In contrast, pulling is expressing tentativeness, remarking, for instance, "I cannot be 100 percent certain." In other words, the difference between push and pull is assertiveness versus tentativeness. Of course, the two forces are not mutually exclusive.

A proposition can involve both push and pull, as in the statement, "The virus is highly dangerous (push), it seems (pull)." These ways of operationalizing push and pull illustrate how speculations emerge and function as social acts in times of uncertainty.

The notion of push and pull was also used, but in a different way, by health officials in San Diego County to characterize their health-emergency communication. Briggs and Hallin (2016) showed that the officials described two opposing modes of interaction with journalists: disseminating official messages (push) versus responding to journalists' inquiries (pull). The push efforts included holding press conferences and creating press releases. The officials admitted that push campaigns are usually funding-driven, as in the case of the amounts of airtime and newspaper space that are provided for disseminating health messages. The pull strategies were exemplified by the classification of reporters' inquiries from "routine, non-controversial, and relatively non-technical" inquiries to "the most potentially explosive issues" that required high-ranking officials' participation (Briggs & Hallin, 2016, p. 56). Under this model of push and pull, the officials revealed their mixed feelings toward the media, viewing journalists as simultaneously important and problematic. Media partnerships can help health officials reach the public with their messages, but the media's goals of selling newspaper or television advertising through sensationalism are fundamentally different from health officials'.

These two models of push and pull primarily concern the characteristics of official communication. There exists a third use of push and pull. In a more balanced view of the push and pull between officials and journalists, Blumler and Esser (2019) discussed the mediatization of politics. They drew on the example of the 2015 UK general election campaign to illustrate two perspectives: media actor-centric versus political actor-centric. On the one hand, the media actor-centric perspective highlights push forces of mediatization, which manifest as a proactive and interventionist reporting style. For example, push forces are realized in at least five types of questions used by journalists to target assertiveness ("Aren't you putting the union at risk?"), adversariness ("You seem to be making all sorts of promises … Aren't you living in a world of fantasy promises?"), accountability ("Why won't you tell them?"), threat to public image ("Why should the voters trust you?"), and challenging an answer (Politician: "I'm confident that can be achieved." Journalist: "'Confidence' is not a 'commitment'?"). On the other hand, the political actor-centric perspective underscores pull strategies of mediatization, which integrate media logic into the political world to facilitate the achievement of political goals. These strategies include news management, media appearances, centralized campaign management, opposition research, and rapid response. Some of these strategies also work in the context of health crisis communication. For instance, news management is about tailoring messages for media consumption and broader public reach by smoothly and articulately responding to events, countering criticisms, and answering challenging questions.

Four Discursive Processes of the Push and Pull

These three different interpretations of the push and pull between government officials and media professionals highlight the lack of scholarly consensus that surrounds this topic. Adopting an integrated approach, in this chapter, I view *push* as journalists' attempt to press officials into addressing newsworthy categories that sensationalize public concerns and *pull* as officials' attempt to pull the focus back to their ways of operationalizing categories in biomedical classifications. This chapter illustrates how this interpretation of push and pull operates within four discursive processes that I identified in the recordings of COVID-19 press conferences. Table 2.1 shows the four processes.

The first two processes are push forces that empower journalists to take a more enterprising role in the production of news information. Disjunctive questions constrain responses by reducing a complex pandemic phenomenon to a choice of two polar-opposite categories, such as mild or severe symptoms. The simplification tends toward controversial and sensational categories. In Mandarin Chinese, disjunctive questions can be presented in one of at least two forms: verb-not-verb (V-not-V) or A-or-B. Each form sets up an action agenda (Clayman & Heritage, 2002) by narrowly defining the appropriate responses. Of course, questions by journalists often do not stand alone; instead, they are asked in particular contexts. Questions may be prefaced or postfaced by metadiscursive framing as part of journalists' exercising greater initiative. For example, a question may be prefaced or postfaced by a third party's opinion to legitimize the questioning—e.g., 國內有醫學專家他們說 'Domestic medical experts are saying'—which in turn intensifies the push forces on the officials to directly respond to the confrontational question.

The pull efforts by health officials are primarily manifested in two discursive processes. One process is delineating categorical relationships in a classification system that entails criteria and examples. The system is used to understand a pandemic phenomenon, such as the definitions of community spread and community-acquired infection when there are individuals in the community who are infected by the virus. Delineating the categories inevitably requires a discussion about who has the power to produce or challenge a classification, to foster or impede the circulation of the classification, and to uphold or

Table 2.1 Four discursive processes of the push and pull

Journalistic push	1	Disjunctive questions erase categorical entanglements and create newsworthiness.
	2	Metadiscursive framing inscribes journalistic initiative into interaction.
Official pull	3	Biocommunicable relationships are recalibrated to emphasize officials' authority and credibility.
	4	Multimodal signs synchronize with speech to objectify biomedical phenomena and reify subject positions.

resist the classification. The scale of these biocommunicable relationships can range from profession ("epidemiologists"), to institution ("WHO"), and to nation ("China"). As such, delineating categorical relationships often involves appealing to authority and building credibility. Finally, the pull efforts are also materialized in the process of using multimodal resources, such as gestures, to transform abstract or invisible pandemic phenomena into discursive objects for public scrutiny. In the process, subjective positions such as those of government officials, health journalists, and the public are foregrounded to make salient who is responsible for which account.

By applying the push-and-pull model in this chapter, I hope to provide a more nuanced understanding of how participants in question-and-answer sessions hosted as part of the Taiwanese COVID-19 press conferences drew on multimodal resources to push forward and pull back their interpretations of classifications. Furthermore, the analysis contributes to journalism literature by showing how public online viewers in Taiwan interpreted the push and pull between officials and journalists and whether push and pull interactions shaped public reception of pandemic classifications. The examples analyzed in this chapter are from three critical moments during the initial outbreak of COVID-19 in early 2020.

Context

My analysis focuses on three key "firsts" in Taiwan—i.e., the first confirmed case, the first community-acquired infection, and the first death—announced by Taiwanese public health officials in January and February 2020. At the time, Taiwan was succeeding in keeping nearly all COVID-19 cases offshore through early and quick border control. While enacting this border control enabled Taiwan to sidestep large outbreaks, the three first-time cases posed threats to the community. Each first-time case indicated a further encroachment of the virus, thus increasing the pressure on officials to closely monitor the situation and continually communicate with the public about the government's preparedness. When talking to the media and the public, the officials had to clearly articulate their classification of each case so as to build a consensus about the status of the crisis and mobilize community cooperation. The focus of each classification differed because each first-time case was unique in context and severity.

The first confirmed case of COVID-19 was announced on January 21, 2020. The person infected with the virus was a Taiwanese businessperson who had traveled back to Taiwan from Wuhan, China, then ground zero of the COVID-19 outbreak, the previous day. The businessperson was stopped at a quarantine site at Taiwan Taoyuan International Airport and was transferred to a hospital for testing and treatment. While there was no risk to the community because the businessperson did not enter the community and was treated at the hospital, controversy brewed when a news report revealed that the businessperson had traveled back to Taiwan despite showing symptoms of a cough and a sore throat while in China. At the press conference announcing the first Taiwanese case of COVID-19, officials emphasized that the businessperson voluntarily disclosed her symptoms to the airline and airport staff. However, viewers online criticized the businessperson for returning to Taiwan knowing that she had such symptoms. BBC News summarized public online criticism on social media: 她堅持搭機回到台灣，使途中和她所接觸的人暴露在感染風險中，是很自私的行為。 'Her insistence on taking the plane back to Taiwan put the people with whom she came into contact at risk of infection. This is a selfish act' (T.-H. Lee, 2020). There were also inconsistencies in the narratives presented by the officials and the businessperson as to whether the businessperson had had a fever before boarding. These inconsistencies weakened public trust in the officials and the businessperson (Lee, 2024a). The fever became a focus because, at that time, there was a lack of knowledge about COVID-19, including whether the disease was similar to SARS, which in earlier years had been shown to be transmissible only after symptoms appeared in those infected. Due to the limited knowledge of COVID-19 at the time and the public criticism of the businessperson's decision to travel when she had symptoms, understanding the medical condition of the first case became a newsworthy topic for journalists to pursue at press conferences. Categories such as severe or mild symptoms needed to be elaborated to help the public understand the disease and assess the ethics of traveling with symptoms.

The first community-acquired infection was ultimately conflated with the first death. When the first death was announced on February 16, 2020, not only had a family member of the deceased been infected with the virus, but also the deceased had had no recent history of international travel. This suggested to many individuals, including Taiwanese public health officials, that undetected virus transmission might have occurred within the community. The deceased was a taxi driver who showed symptoms at the end of January, was hospitalized in early February, and passed away in the hospital on February 15. It was not until after the taxi driver's death that officials received medical confirmation that the cause of death had been COVID-19. When an official announced the first death and explained the abrupt timeline from symptom appearance to death, it immediately sparked a wave of shock and panic among the public: How could the deadly virus have silently infiltrated Taiwan with its strict border control? In light of the first death, the officials classified the crisis status of Taiwan as 社區感染 'community infection,' which denoted the location of the infection, and rejected journalists' use of the term 社區傳播 'community spread,' which denoted widespread infection in the community. The journalists challenged the official classification by relaying the voices of other social pundits and the US Centers for Disease Control and Prevention, which classified Taiwan's status as one of community spread (Lee, 2024b). The officials scrambled to investigate the death in the following days. On February 20, 2020, health officials announced in the daily press conference that the taxi driver very likely had been infected by one of his passengers, who had returned to Taiwan from China where there were large outbreaks of COVID-19 in early 2020. This piece of evidence was used to support the official classification of community infection because the infection source was traceable. The episode illustrates the process of (de)constructing categories as evidence was being uncovered by retracing infection sources.

Throughout the press conferences centered on the three first times, health officials and journalists engaged in the push and pull of negotiating classifications. Figure 2.1 illustrates the typical corporeal participation framework (De León, 2011) of such a conference. A panel of officials is onstage, whereas journalists are offstage. This spatial arrangement creates a participation framework of two primary groups (i.e., officials and journalists) and orients both groups toward a face-to-face exchange. Interactional sequences are primarily regimented by the onstage panel as the officials allocate turns to offstage journalists one at a time during the question-and-answer session. Journalists have to bid for the official permission to speak. They also need to ask all of their questions upon being selected. As such, journalists cannot immediately follow up on official responses. Additionally, each official's institutional identity is made visible through not only the nameplates on the table but also the seating arrangement. That is, the commander takes the central seat, and his executive officer and an expert on infectious diseases (known as the convenor) flank the commander. Thus, the corporeal participation framework of the conference embodies institutional power and prescribes interactional norms.

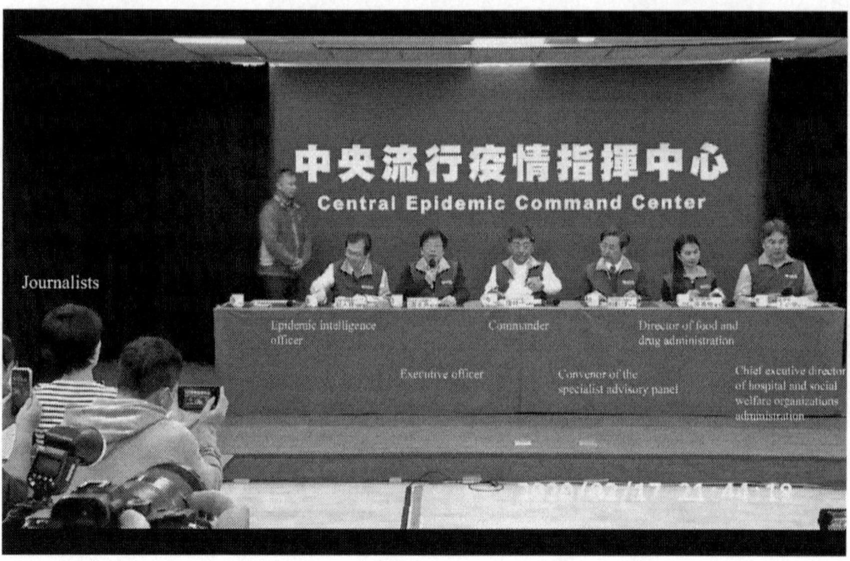

Figure 2.1 Corporeal participation framework in the press conference.

Source: Taiwan Centers for Disease Control, February 17, 2020. www.youtube.com/watch?v=Ce3DJoHHsOM

Health officials were believed to be the sole producers of health information and knowledge. They collected and analyzed crisis information prior to each press conference and then disseminated the knowledge at the press conference. However, upon studying the participation framework of the press conferences, it becomes clear that journalists played an equally important role in the production of biomedical objects and subjects.

To understand the coproduction process, I identified sequences that involved negotiations of pandemic classifications. These sequences occurred during the question-and-answer sessions of the various conferences. In what follows, I analyze how the sequences were initiated by journalists; how the journalists framed their questions and relayed public concerns; how officials responded to the questions; and how the officials' speech co-occurred with the use of multimodal signs such as artifacts, gestures, eye gaze, and bodily orientation.

Analysis

This section presents an analysis of the question-and-answer sequences between health journalists and officials. These sequences are organized into two sections: the medical condition of the first case and the crisis status of the community (i.e., the first community-acquired infection and the first death). At the end of the section about the first case, I triangulate comments made by online viewers with the interactional analysis. In the section about the community status, I present the triangulation after the analysis of each sequence because the online live-chat comments are about specific speech practices at the conferences.

The Medical Condition of the First Case

The first Taiwanese case of COVID-19 garnered much public attention not only because it resurfaced the distressing memory of 2003 SARS epidemic, which had also first broken out in Taiwan as a result of a Taiwanese businessperson traveling home from China (Wang et al., 2003), but also because it stirred an ethical controversy regarding the businessperson's awareness of her symptoms before traveling. The public was keen to know the similarities and differences between SARS and COVID-19, the seriousness of the symptoms, and the scale of the outbreak inside and outside China. Journalists played an important role in seeking the answers to these questions.

Rather than simply transmitting information produced by health officials, Taiwanese journalists proceeded to present polarized categories and to push for revealing responses. This way of "preformulating" (Jacobs, 1999, p. xii) newsworthy categories is associated in the dataset with the use of disjunctive questions. Excerpt 1 shows how a journalist used the polarized A-or-B disjunctive question 輕症還是重症 'mild or severe' to present newsworthy categories as biomedical objects, only to subsequently adopt the open-ended question of 怎麼樣 'how' to give officials latitude in developing their responses (1). Newsworthiness and neutralism were delicately woven into the question design.

Excerpt 1

1	Journalist	uh想請問她現在顯示病症是輕症還是重症, 現在..狀況怎麼樣.	Uh, (I) would like to ask if her symptoms appear to be mild or severe. How is (she doing) now?
2	Medical officer	...(2.6)呃=, ..依據世界衛生組織在一月= 十幾號公布的-- 就是暫時的指引那,	Uh, according to the temporary guidelines published by World Health Organization in the middle of January,
3		..呃= 呃=這個-我們英文叫severe pneumonia, 欸=也就是呃比較嚴重的肺炎.	uh uh in English, we call this 'severe pneumonia.' Uh that is rather severe pneumonia.
4		..那這個嚴重的定義是第一個他沒有用<L氧氣的時候L>, 嗯就是他會需要用氧氣, ..呃才能夠維持到那個=呃=呃=, ..呼吸的正常的血氧濃度.	So the definition of severe is first when they are not on oxygen- Uh that is, they will need to be on oxygen .. uh in order to maintain that- uh uh .. normal oxygen saturation (levels) of breathing.
5		第二個就是他的, ..呼吸的速度會比較快.	The second is their .. respiratory rate will be faster.
6		那這個病人因為她還需要用=, ..就是在鼻子上掛著=, ..掛著氧氣駒,	So this patient- because she still needs to use, .. that is on (her) nose, .. wearing oxygen (tubes).

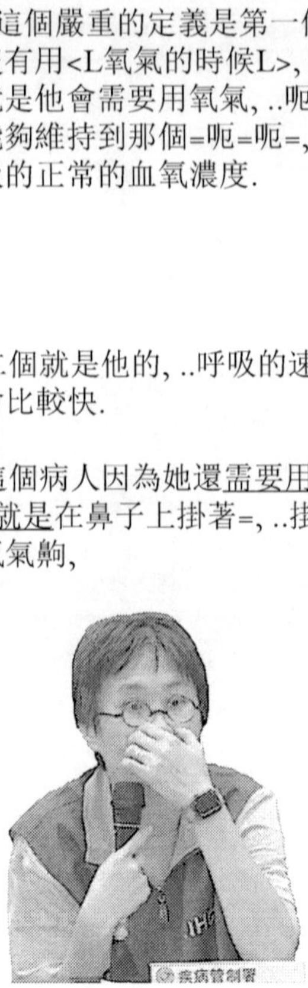

7		呃所以依照這個=, 呃= 分類呢, ..呃 我們是把它叫做嚴重的肺炎.	Uh so according to this, uh classification, .. uh we call it severe pneumonia.
8		那-, 當然她目前沒有要使用呼吸器或是什麼的狀況.	Then, of course she is currently not in a condition needing to use a ventilator or that kind of thing

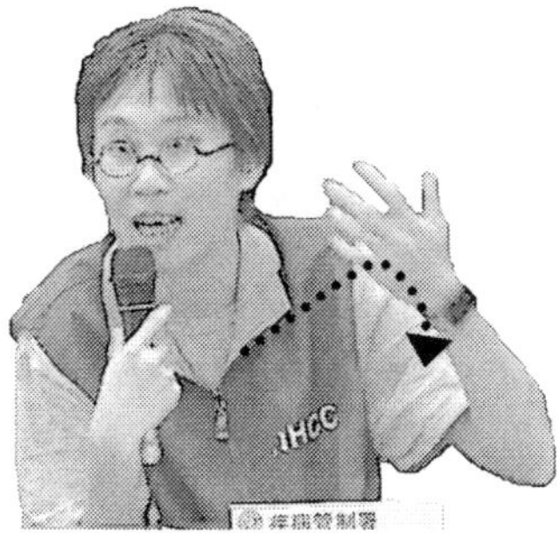

In Excerpt 1, following the journalist's queries, the medical officer recalibrated the diagnostic category of 嚴重 'severity.' She began by citing the authoritative third party of 世界衛生組織 the 'World Health Organization' (2) and adopted the English medical category "severe pneumonia" (3) to underscore the original term in medicine, thereby establishing her credibility. Subsequently, she introduced two criteria and explained how the case met one of the criteria. Gestures—an icon (6) that visualized and a beat (8) that emphasized the medical condition of the patient—were recruited to visually depict why the case fell into the WHO's category of severity, which did not align with the lay understanding of the word 嚴重 'severe.' Ultimately, Excerpt 1 demonstrates how the journalist recruited the use of a polar disjunctive question to pursue categories of interest whereas the official recontextualized "severe" within the biomedical diagnosis of severe pneumonia.

While disjunctive questions have an action agenda, when a response rejects both candidate answers without elaboration, journalists' discontent is on display. Excerpt 2 is a case in point.

Excerpt 2

1	Journalist	那名台商是重症還是輕症, 從臨床判斷.	Are the Taiwanese businessperson's symptoms severe or mild, clinically diagnosed?

2	Medical officer	唔=, ...(1.1)她不是輕症.	Ah, … (her symptoms) are not mild
3		呃=, 她=也不是到插管的重症, 嗯.	Uh, (her symptoms) are also not severe to require intubation, mh.
4		…@@<P uh P>,	
5	All	(Laughter)	

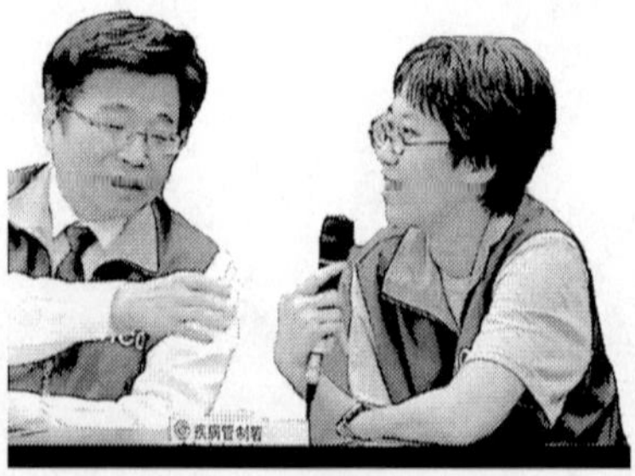

6	Commander	不是X, ..今天被<MRC確診MRC>, ..她就是我們所謂的<MRC 嚴重肺炎 MRC>.	No X, today having been confirmed (as a COVID-19 case), .. she is the so-called (having) severe pneumonia.
7		...(.7)齁啊只是在<MRC嚴重肺炎裡面MRC>, ...那今天觀察到的,	Okay, ah but in severe pneumonia, … and what has been observed today,

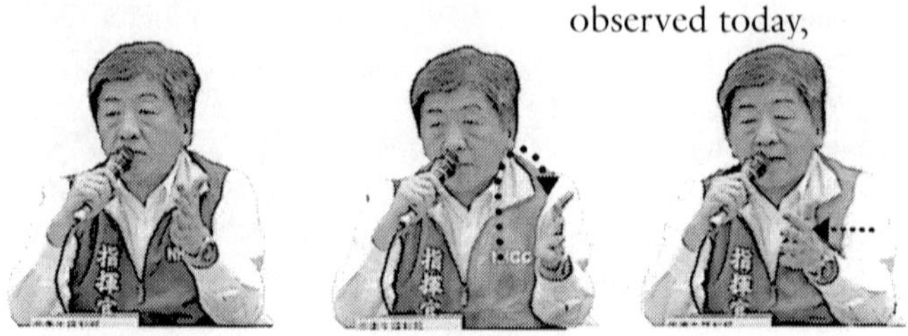

8		就是說燒已經在退了, ..那也沒有到插管的情況,	is that, (her) fever is subsiding, .. and (her symptoms) did not get to the condition of (requiring) intubation.

9	...夠所以不是在嚴重肺炎<L裡面的重症L>.	Okay so not severe symptoms in severe pneumonia.

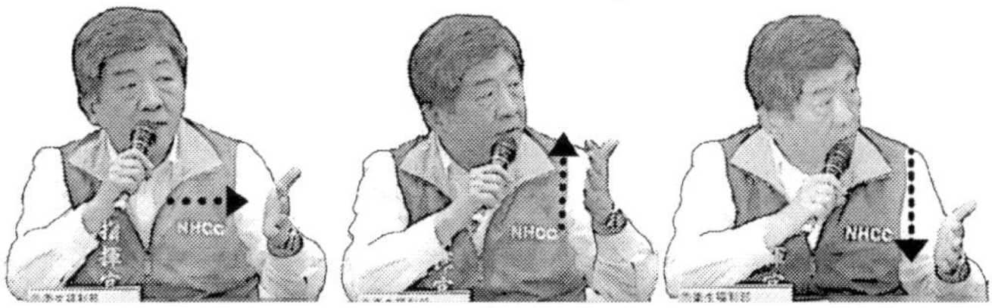

As shown in Excerpt 2, following a request to clarify their question, the journalist launched the polar disjunctive question of 重症還是輕症 'severe or mild.' The agenda of the question was metadiscursively tightened by the post-positioned statement 從臨床判斷 'clinically diagnosed' that blocked all answers other than a biomedical interpretation. Nevertheless, the medical officer rejected both options with hesitation as shown in her fillers 唔 'Ah' and 呃 'Uh,' as well as her use of elongation and long pauses (2–4). This rejection resulted in awkward laughter among all individuals, including the officer herself. The executive officer attempted to intervene by brusquely reaching over to grab the microphone from the medical officer (5).

The commander eventually took the floor to repair the mishap by complicating the categorical dichotomy of mild versus severe. He first stated that any confirmed case was classified as 嚴重肺炎 'severe pneumonia' (6). He then explained health officials' observation in relation to the category of severe pneumonia. As he was explaining the degree of severity presented by the pneumonia, in line 7, a small arc was formed by his gesture (left hand opened, fingers extended, and palm facing his right) and forearm movement (up and then down). The creation of this arc was synchronized with his speech of 嚴重肺炎裡面 'in severe pneumonia.' Subsequently, his forearm moved horizontally from his left to right, which overlapped with the speech 今天觀察到的 'what has been observed today' (7). His gestures and forearm movements thus created vector spaces that illustrated the degree of severity of the pneumonia. The status of the patient was close to the center of his body where the severe symptoms indicated by 燒已經在退了 'fever is subsiding' and 那也沒有到插管的情況 'did not get to the condition of requiring intubation' were absent (8). To illustrate the opposite side of the vector, in line 9, his forearm moved from his central body toward his left. This movement showing that distant to his central body are those severe symptoms associated with the category of severe pneumonia. The up and down beats emphasized the severity of the category. Overall, the gesture vector constructed through the horizontal and vertical motions of the forearm worked in tandem with speech to transform biomedical objects from a conceptual category to a visual representation.

A gesture vector is equally important in Excerpt 3, which illustrates journalists and officials discussing the nationality of the first person diagnosed with COVID-19.

Excerpt 3

1.	Journalist	我想確認一下喔, ..所以這一位女台商是不是全球, ..現在知道, ..uh中國籍以外的第一位...病例.	I would like to confirm. .. So is this female Taiwanese businessperson … the first case in the world, .. known at present, ..uh not of Chinese nationality?
2	Executive officer	...(1.4)中國以外的病例,	…A case outside China.
3	Journalists	中國籍以外.	Not of Chinese nationality.
4	Executive officer	..中國籍以外的病例,	A case not of Chinese nationality.
5	All	[@@@@@]	
6	Executive officer	[欸=]好像其他的--	Uhm it seems other-
7	Epidemic intelligence officer	...(1.6)不太清楚他[[的..其它國籍]],	(it is) not clear about their- .. other nationalities,
8	Executive officer	[[不太清楚其他國家的那個國]]籍[嘿].	not clear about the nationalities of other countries' (cases), mh.
9	Epidemic intelligence officer	[對].	Right.
10		...(2.1)日方那個,	The one in Japan-
11	XXX((audience))	…你想太多了.	…You think too much.
12	Executive officer	...(.7)嘿因為=...泰國的話他們是宣布很清楚嘛,	…Mh because … in the case of Thailand, they announce (it) very clearly.
13		..就是說=, 他們好像是=, ..是=陸--..<u>大陸的國籍</u>, ..<u>中國籍</u>.	That is, they seem to be, be Main- ..Mainland nationality, .. Chinese nationality.

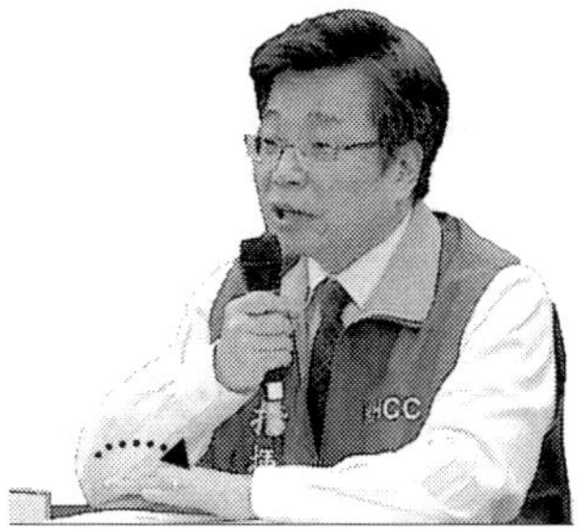

14	...<A那陸方的那個的部分的話, 我們沒有看到他正式的文件裡頭A>, 是敘述哪一個國籍嘿.	As for the part (about cases) on the Mainland, we have not seen in their official document stating which nationalities, mh.

In Excerpt 3, the journalist recruited the verb of saying 確認 'confirm' to introduce a V-not-V disjunctive question 是不是 (1). The newsworthy potential of the question lies in two aspects: (1) to infer whether the virus had spread outside China, then the ground-zero of the pandemic; and (2) to invoke categories that implicate Taiwan's enduring struggle with China over Taiwan's sovereignty, particularly when Taiwan's ruling government was believed to have alienated Taiwan from China. The sequence thus demonstrates how classifications inevitably involve power maneuvers at broader institutional, geopolitical, and historical levels.

After negotiating his understanding of the question (1–5), the executive officer turned to the other officers on the panel. The intelligence officer stepped in to answer the question by stating that health officials did not have the information, which the executive officer echoed (7–9). Subsequently, the executive officer cited the third party 泰國 'Thailand' and adopted the declarative verb 宣布 'announced' modified by the degree adverb 很 'very' and evaluative adjective 清楚 'clearly,' which allowed him to evade the journalist's attempt to steer the sequence toward other cross-Strait issues (12). As he shared the information about the Chinese national in Thailand, his fingers moved outward to indicate this case was external to Thailand (13). Toward the end, the executive officer invoked the institutional 我們 'we' to indicate that health officials in Taiwan had not seen relevant information in China's official documents (14). This indication was subtle in the sense that it contrasted with his earlier description of Thailand as a country that discloses its information 很清楚 'very clearly.' It also indirectly echoed the international criticism of China's lack of transparency in updating pandemic information.

Online viewers left comments beneath the YouTube video that included the sequences presented in Excerpts 1–3. The comments offer a glimpse into what pandemic information was received. For example, despite the officials' subtleties in handling cross-Strait issues at the press conferences, the online comments explicitly or sarcastically created subjective positions that targeted cross-Strait relationships, such as 'A hernia epidemic from the ancestral land,' in which the commenter borrowed the register of the Chinese government to reference China as the ancestral land of Taiwan. Additionally, fever was not simply a biomedical category but part of a conspiracy: 'Currently, internal confidential documents in China reveal that this atypical pneumonia may not cause fever, so it may be useless to screen [people] by body-temperature measurement.' A linear biocommunicable model of transmitting health information from officials to the public cannot account for how health information circulates here (see also Briggs & Hallin, 2016). The online commenters attempted to interpret the medical condition of the first case through the lens of cross-Strait politics. In an era of livestreamed press conferences, public online engagement in the production and circulation of crisis classifications becomes simultaneously a problem for and a solution to making pandemic categories travel broadly.

The Status of the Community

About a month after the detection of the first COVID-19 case, the virus infiltrated Taiwan. Much of the ensuing discussion revolved around the meanings of 社區感染 'community-acquired infection' and 社區傳播 'community spread' as the controversy about how to interpret the ramifications of the first death intensified. The controversy came to dominate the question-and-answer sessions during the daily press conferences as more details about the first death were uncovered, including the victim's lack of recent documented international travel. Excerpt 4 is an example in which a journalist recruited other pundits to push the official to classify the crisis situation.

Excerpt 4

1	Journalist	然後也想請教, ..我國目前的疫情大概是處於, ..圍堵期還是已經=, ..進入了減災期,	And also (I) would like to ask, .. is the pandemic status of our nation roughly in, .. containment phase or has it already, .. entered mitigation phase?
2		因為今天早上有學者, ..呃=有在討論這兩個-- ..這兩個疫情是有不同的學校的防疫措施,	Because this morning there were scholars, ..uh discussing these two- .. these two (phases of) pandemic status have different pandemic-control measures at schools.

3		..也希望中央能夠=, 呃回應, ..謝謝.	Also hope the central (government) can, uh respond. .. Thanks.
4		((several turns about response to other questions omitted))	
5	Executive officer	...(4.4)我想是-- 您剛才所提到是現在是在減災期還是圍堵期,	... I think (it) is- you just mentioned about if at the moment (we) are in the phase of mitigation or containment.
6		我那個-- ..這有一點可以最容易看得出來,	I the- .. there is one thing that is the easiest telling (feature).
7		我們檢疫有沒有放鬆, ...我們檢疫現在一點都沒有放鬆,	Have we relaxed our quarantine (measures)? ... Our quarantine measures at the moment are not relaxed at all
8		..但是呢我也可以跟大家報告, ...我們也為了後續, 疫情的發展,	But I can also report to everyone, ... we also, for the subsequent development of the pandemic,
9		齁都會想定大概比較不好的狀況預作準備,	okay (we) will consider probably worse scenarios and prepare in advance.
10		..比如講說, ...我們預計,	..Say for example, ... we estimate,
11		啊如果是清空病床要怎麼樣子清空, 齁他的順序是怎麼樣, ..哪一些優先, ..哪個地區是怎麼樣,	ah if freeing up hospital beds, how to free them up. Mh what will be the sequence? .. Which ones have priority? .. How it will be? Which areas?
12		..所以說我們目前的處理的情形, 齁還是--..應該是蠻清楚的啦.	..So the current situation of our handling, mh still is- .. should be quite clear.

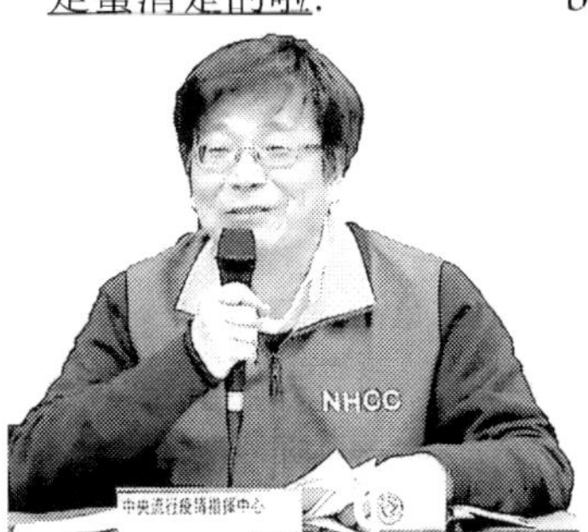

In Excerpt 4, the journalist launched a disjunctive question (1) to press the officials to identify the community's current phase (i.e., containment or mitigation). The questioning was amplified by invoking knowledgeable pundits, 學者 'scholars,' in a post-positioned statement (2). This invocation neutralized the journalist's push because the journalist was relaying the content of pundits' discussions. Rather than responding to the action agenda prescribed by the journalist's questioning (i.e., selecting an A or B response), the executive officer reframed the question by introducing a criterion in the superlative 最容易 'the easiest' (6) and adopting a V-not-V disjunctive question 有沒有 'have or have not' (7). His response to the reframed question was an explicit negation coupled with the intensifier 一點都沒有 'not at all' (7). Through list construction (11), he enumerated provisional plans for a worst-case scenario. In the end, he returned to responding to the question about the crisis status. His allusion to the containment phase (i.e., no community spread) was expressed through a constellation of the temporal adverb 還是 'still,' the obligatory modal verb 應該 'should,' the degree adverb 蠻 'quite,' and the contextualization cue (Gumperz, 1988) of his smiling face (12).

The push and pull of public-health information in Excerpt 4 was well received by online viewers. These viewers offered a positive assessment of the journalist's ways of speaking 'Talking is really clear and polite'; content of the questions 'Right, isn't it very good to ask what the public wants to know?'; and affiliation 'Mandarin Daily News very clearly focuses on education-related questions.' The viewers made a similarly positive assessment of the officer 'Executive Officer Chou is also very steady.' Thus, Excerpt 4 illustrates that when classification questions are appropriately framed and justified, officials' responses are more likely to be well received by the public, even if the officials do not directly respond to the classification questions.

In contrast to the implicit deflection seen in Excerpt 4, at times officials redirected the focus back to their message by explaining the criteria behind their classifications, as shown in Excerpt 5.

Excerpt 5

1	Journalist	因為我們證實現在已經有社區感染了,	Because we confirmed that there is already community-acquired infection,
2		那..是可以說=, ..<MRC本土= ..感染嗎?MRC>..還是只是本土死亡案例而已.	then.. is it ok to say, .. local infection? .. Or is it only a case of local death?
3	Commander	((Several turns about responding to other questions omitted))	

4	那剛剛再問到社區齁(TSK), 基本上社區傳播的一個..定義齁?	Mh just a moment ago (a journalist) asked about community again mh. Basically a definition .. of community spread.
5	..齁它一個定義就是說社區活--	Mh one of its definitions is that community acti-
6	在社區裡面走就有感染的風險.	There is a risk of infection just by walking in the community.
7	...齁那, 通常齁它有幾樣的徵兆, 齁專業上來講,	..Mh uh, usually mh it has several kinds of signs, mh professionally speaking.

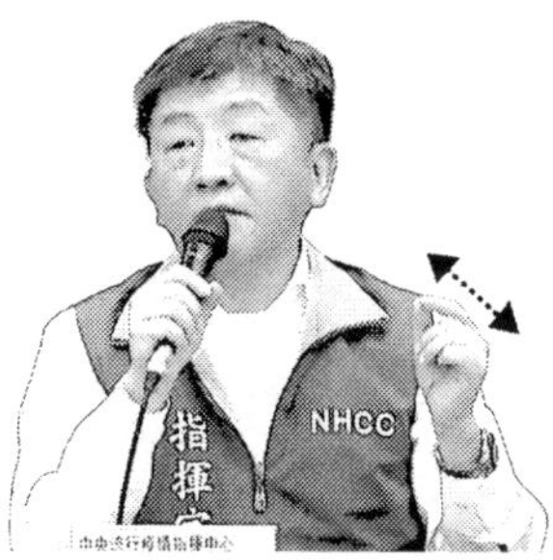

8	..一個是確定病例無法找出<L感染來源L>.	One is being unable to find the infection source of a confirmed case.
9	就跟我們今天,	Just like us today
10	目前的情況..是一樣的,	The current situation .. is the same.
11	..然後第二個是,	Then the second one is,
12	..本地感染的個案, 已遠超過, ...境外移入感染的個案數.	the cases of local infection, already far exceed … the number of cases from abroad.
13	那這沒-這沒有,	Mh this is not- this is not (the case).

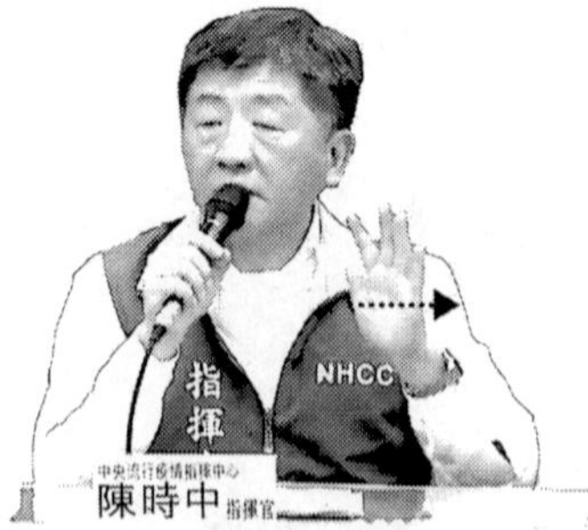

14	..齁我們基本上大部分都是境外..移入的個案數.	Mh we basically the majority of cases are all from .. abroad.
15	...(.7)然後第三個已經出現, ..持-持續性或連續性的一個傳播鏈.	Then the third one, there is already, .. a conti- continuous or successive chain of infection.
16	..齁就一傳十十傳百,	Mh, like, one spreads to ten. Ten spread to one hundred.

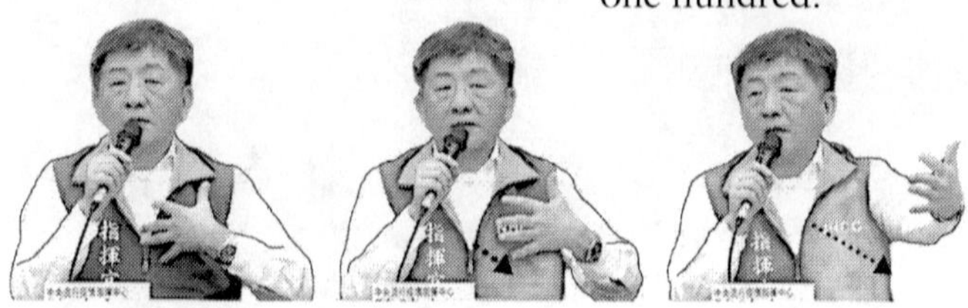

17	..齁臺灣也沒有這個情況.	Mh Taiwan has no such scenario either.

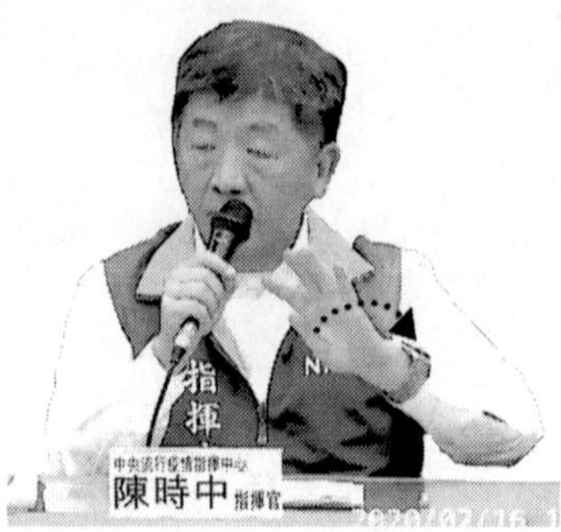

18	..然後第四個是說, ..廣泛地發生有群聚的事件.	Then the fourth one is that there are widespread occurrences of cluster (infection) incidents.

19	..<u>臺灣也沒有</u>.	Taiwan has none either.
	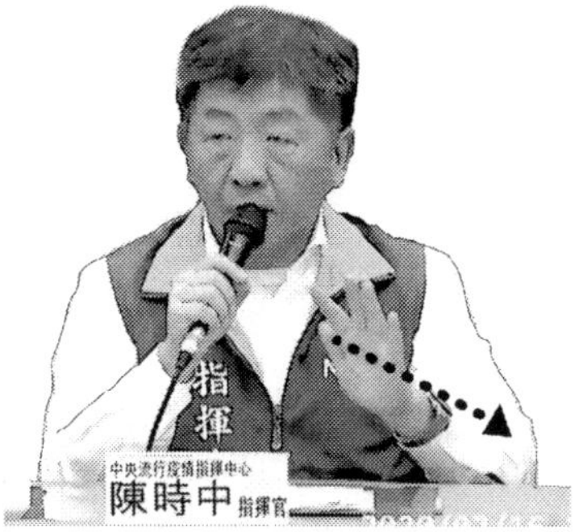	
20	...齁所以我們講說社區傳播, 我們現在這是一個--有這樣的一個徵兆跟警訊,	Mh so we say that community spread. We are now- this is a- there is this kind of sign and warning.

Excerpt 5 shows that in a prefatory statement, the journalist put forward the category of community-acquired infection as a presumptive foundation. This presumption was created through the generic collectivity 我們 'we' and the verb of saying 證實 'confirmed' (1), which showed an attempt to neutralize and legitimate the question. Following the preface, a yes-or-no question was combined with the disjunctive question 還是 'or' to drive the officials to disclose whether the first death had been deemed a case of local infection or local death (2). Embedding the attitudinal adverb 只是 'only' in the question, the journalist suggested that local infection was more serious than local death.

In response, the commander prefaced the criteria for assessing whether community spread was happening. In line 7, the preface was metadiscursively framed with the phrase 專業上來講 'professionally speaking' and imagistically highlighted through his precision-grip gestures (thumb to tip of forefinger) that had a focus effect on making sharp, effective points (Lempert, 2011). Each criterion then unfolded in the interface of speech and gestures. Particularly important is a gesture vector created to illustrate a continuous transmission chain (16). Illustrating this biomedical object, the commander's speech focused on the scale of case multiplication (i.e., one, ten, one hundred) while his left forearm extended outward to metaphorically visualize the scale. With a single exception, the criteria were considered inapplicable to classify Taiwan as an instance of community spread because Taiwan does not meet the criteria. The inapplicability was explicitly rejected through the negation marker 沒有 'not,' coupled with emblematic gestures (13, 17, 19). To encapsulate his main message, the commander related his classifications of the current status as a 一個徵兆跟警訊 'sign and warning' of community spread (20). In other words, the status of Taiwan had yet to reach community spread.

The journalist's question was criticized by online viewers because they considered the question to have been answered earlier during the conference: 'if there is no question, stop seeking attention. Journalist'; 'not yet. The journalist can't understand'; and 'Stop asking idiot questions … China Times.' In contrast to the comments bluntly criticizing the journalist, the only comment on the commander's explanation blended endearment (referencing the commander's first name) and power (framing his talk as instruction): 'instruction by Shih-chung.'

As more details of contact tracing were unveiled to suggest that the first victim had contracted the virus in Taiwan, journalists became hostile toward officials' evasiveness (Excerpt 6).

Excerpt 6

1	Journalist	..可不可以請..部長, ..<L明確地說=L>, ..我們今天公布的這兩個確診的案例, ...是不是代表有社區感染,	May (I) please ask the minister .. to clearly say, if the two confirmed cases that we announced today mean that there is community-acquired infection.
2		如果是就說是, 如果說不是就說不是, 謝謝.	If yes, just say yes. If no, just say no. Thanks.
3	Commander	...(.7)那昨天為了這個問題就弄到很晚齁,	Uh because of this question, yesterday (we) finished very late mh.
4		((several turns about responding to other questions omitted))	
5		..那我想這還是, 齁維持說-應該是說一個零星的, ..齁個案在社區內受到感染.	Mh I think this is still, mh maintain it as- should say a sporadic .. mh case infected in the community.
6		...(1.7)那剛剛有問到那些齁, ..社區感染,	And just a moment ago, (some) asked those mh .. community-acquired infection.
7		請問那個-路-這路徑齁,	Asked the- path- the pathway mh.

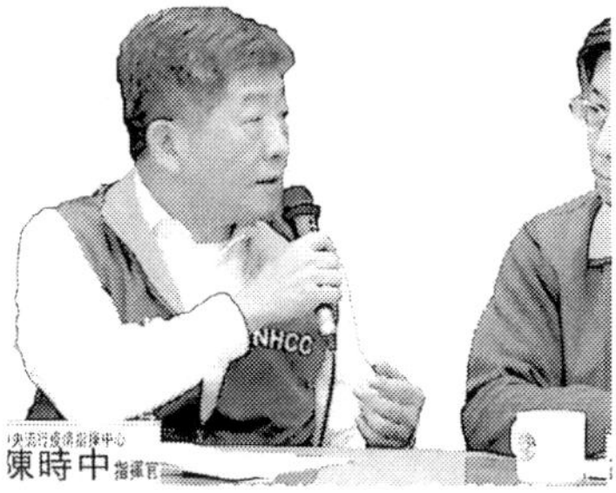

8 是不是要<X讓X>張教授來補充. Should (we) ask Professor Chang to supplement (other information)?

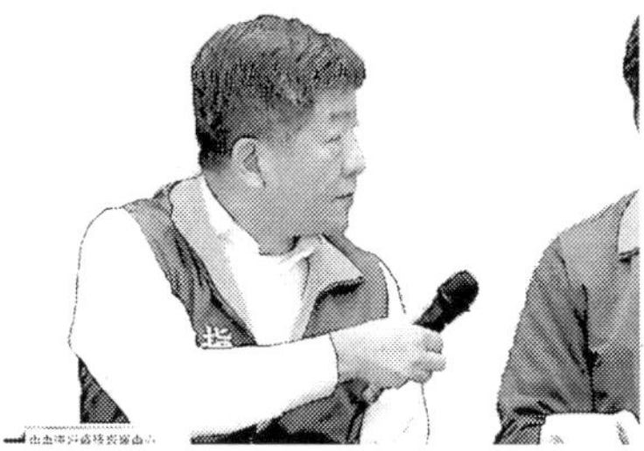

In Excerpt 6, the gravity of the question was revealed in the journalist's use of two V-not-V disjunctive questions, 可不可以 and 是不是 (1). The metadiscursive framing of the questions 明確地說 'clearly say' (1) further delimited the manner and explicitly constrained the response options: 如果是就說是, 如果說不是就說不是 'If yes, just say yes. If no, just say no' (2). This ultimately pedagogicalized the question-and-answer sequence.

Instead of continuing the pedagogical footing, the commander resisted the action agenda (i.e., responding with yes or no). In line 5, he recruited the subjective epistemic claim 我想 'I think,' the obligatory modal verb 應該 'should,' and the verb of saying 說 'say' to classify the case as a 零星的 'sporadic' infection within the community. To clarify the category 社區感染 'community-acquired infection' raised again by the journalist, he allocated the turn to another panelist physically (orienting and leaning toward the panelist) and linguistically (evoking the category of a knowledgeable expert, a 教授 'professor; 7–8). Notice that rather than using the second-person pronoun "you" as in a conversation, the commander referenced a professional identity for the sake of the bystanders, the journalists. This shift of footing demonstrates how health officials modulated their semiotic resources to build up their subjective positions of authority and credibility.

As the sequence in Excerpt 6 unfolded, online viewers lashed out at the journalist for the tone of questioning used: 'It's really impolite'; 'Why is the journalist's attitude so bad?'; and 'something wrong? Sanlih journalist.' No comment was made on the commander's responses.

Discussion

This chapter sought to understand how, during the initial three grim milestones of the pandemic—the first case, the first community-acquired infection, and the first death—classifications were biomediatized at the COVID-19 press conferences in Taiwan. The analysis shows that media and health professionals coproduced biomedical objects and subjects in the push and pull of COVID-19 discourses. On the one hand, journalists exerted their power by launching disjunctive questions in specific metadiscourse frames to "push" officials for elaborations on newsworthy categories. On the other hand, health officials resisted the proposed categories in journalists' questioning. Instead, the officials strove to "pull" the attention back to their classifications by drawing boundaries around their preferred biocommunicable model. For example, the officials referenced the biomedical subjects of institutions ('we'), international organizations ('World Health Organization'), and knowledgeable experts ('Professor Chang) to amplify the authority of their classifications. In witnessing the unfolding of this push and pull, public online viewers, rather than simply passively absorbing health information, engaged in the interactions as arbitrators. The new interactional format of news media (i.e., YouTube live streaming) afforded them space to leave blunt remarks that praised or criticized both parties' speech styles, which, according to an interview study by Chen (2021), threatened journalists' professional engagement during subsequent press conferences.

If classifications are segmentations of the world that aim at maintaining social order (Bowker & Star, 1999), then the push and pull of COVID-19 discourses show that when social order is fraying at the edges, classifications are brought to the foreground as discursive actions for reconceptualizing the nature and retaining social order. At a larger societal scale, such actions socialize individuals into groups that recognize the import of new cultural practices (e.g., social distancing) in light of the crisis in nature. Likewise, classifications may be recruited to resist changes to existing practices, leading to the formation of group identities such as COVID deniers or anti-vaxxers. Classifications thus are integral to group memberships and subjective positions. Categories in classifications are biomediatized objects created through complex interactions in which health officials, journalists, institutions, geopolitical tensions, pathogens, and online viewers are all directly or indirectly implicated.

Turning attention to biocommunicability (Briggs & Hallin, 2016), in the analysis, I uncovered features of language use that reflect the identities of journalists and officials. Journalists pursued newsworthiness through disjunctive questions and displayed their legitimacy, neutralism, and sometimes adversarialness in metadiscursive framing. In contrast, health officials recruited third-party attribution to build up their credibility and authority, list construction to strengthen the appearance of logical reasoning, and gesture vector to illustrate abstract categories. A common tactic adopted by the officials was to address issues raised by the journalists but avoid responding to the corresponding action agendas (an A or B response). This avoidance might be due to the complexity of the pandemic circumstance from the biomedical gaze. However, if action agendas are constantly dismissed, officials may be deemed untrustworthy. While the officials' responses embodied the model of power-biomedical authority, the journalists in all the excerpts analyzed fulfilled their duty of monitoring, detecting, and questioning inconsistencies between official and other discourses. The boundaries between the scenes that unfolded in front of and behind the camera during the live-streamed conferences were blurred (Jacobs, 2011), and power maneuvers were vividly live-streamed. Online comments by public viewers suggest that as the new media discourse of pandemic live-streaming becomes part of everyday life, political motives, conspiracy theories, and geopolitical tensions intrude on the process of disseminating public health information. That is, health information is continuously filtered through online viewers' stances on societal issues such as domestic politics and geopolitical escalations across the Taiwan Strait. Under this influence, images of official and journalistic impartiality are constantly confronted. Politicizing and conspiracizing public health information thwarts efforts to transparently disseminate health information. A lingering task is to maintain an open online platform that provides direct access to health information without being overtaken by an infodemic.

Previous research on press conferences, COVID-19 public health communication, and the intersection of the two has uncovered key rhetorical features of speech (e.g., Bhatia, 2006; Degani, 2022; Vásquez, 2021). This chapter shows that as a speech genre, the press conference entails its own participation framework that is continuously modulated by the interweaving of speech, gesture, eye gaze, facial expression, and bodily orientation. Category biomediatization in this speech genre requires researchers to study delicate power maneuvers in the dynamics of a multi-party participation framework. Even the referential term 'health officials' does not suggest a homogenous group of individuals. Each official on the panel was tasked with a different aspect of pandemic response coordination; their bodily movements and seating arrangement implicated who was permitted to say what to whom. Likewise, while the semiosis of journalists was not broadcasted, the journalists' routine of stating their representative medium before asking questions provided the officials and online viewers with information about whether and, if so, how the given issue of concern was subject to certain ideologies upheld by journalistic affiliations. As such, press conferences are potent sites of knowledge and power wherein individuals recruit semiotic resources to convey concerns and offer assurance.

Implication

The push and pull between officials and journalists can be well managed if several interactional intricacies are taken into account. First, in response to journalists' push for newsworthy categories, officials must be prepared to explain why the categories are (in)adequate for characterizing the crisis status. An effective explanation needs clear criteria and concrete examples to help the public conceptualize the relationship between the crisis situation and the categories. Particularly important is the recognition that although biomedical categories embedded in official accounts may be the same as the vernacular terms used by the public, the categories and terms may not share the same referential meaning. For example, community-acquired infection and community spread were considered by many laypeople to be synonyms but the officials did not see them the same way. When socializing the public to biomedical categories, systematic criteria and concrete examples become even more important. That is, categories need to be contextualized to bring to forefront their precise meanings and achieve public consensus.

Secondly, journalists use disjunctive questions not only to push for sensational categories but also to solicit details from officials. Officials may resist journalists' classification by reframing the disjunctive options (Excerpts 1, 5, and 6). The journalists may also admit their lack of information (Excerpt 3) or suggest a category through implicit inference (Excerpt 4). However, it is considered infelicitous by all parties (Excerpt 2) to directly reject journalists' categories without a detailed explanation. When rejecting journalists' categories, officials should consider proposing categories that more adequately characterize the situation, which provides journalists with the language to report on the crisis. Reframing disjunctive questions is equally important in handling journalists' questions. Not only should the reframing reorient public attention to official classifications, but it should target public viewers by helping them understand the gist and importance of journalistic questioning. Moreover, classification inevitably involves abstract reasoning, particularly in the realm of biomedicine. To ensure official explanation is accessible to the public, a multimodal display of categorical relationships, such as one with gesture vectors, can help unpack the abstractness and foster the public uptake of complex categories.

Finally, while many of the suggestions here are about preparing officials to tackle journalistic questions, the push and pull can be informative and well-received by the public if journalists clearly articulate and persuasively justify their questions by linking their questions to an aspect of public life (see Excerpt 4), which creates opportunities for officials to introduce and elaborate on their classifications. In other words, the push and pull can become a joint endeavor between journalists and officials to help the public understand the crisis and relate classifications.

References

Bhatia, A. (2006). Critical discourse analysis of political press conferences. *Discourse & society*, *17*(2), 173–203. https://doi.org/10.1177/0957926506058057

Blom, J. N., Rønlev, R., Hansen, K. R., & Ljungdalh, A. K. (2021). The potentials and pitfalls of interactional speculations by journalists and experts in the media: The case of Covid-19. *Journalism Studies*, *22*(9), 1142–1160. https://doi.org/10.1080/1461670X.2021.1925950

Blumler, J. G., & Esser, F. (2019). Mediatization as a combination of push and pull forces: Examples during the 2015 UK general election campaign. *Journalism*, *20*(7), 855–872. https://doi.org/10.1177/1464884918754850

Bowker, G. C., & Star, S. L. (1999). *Sorting things out: Classification and its consequences*. MIT Press.

Briggs, C. L. (2011). Biocommunicability. In M. Singer & P. I. Erickson (Eds.), *A companion to medical anthropology* (pp. 459–476). Wiley-Blackwell. https://doi.org/10.1002/9781444395303.ch23

Briggs, C. L., & Hallin, D. C. (2016). *Making health public: How news coverage is remaking media, medicine, and contemporary life*. Routledge. https://doi.org/10.4324/9781315658049

Briggs, C. L., & Mantini-Briggs, C. (2016). *Tell me why my children died: Rabies, indigenous knowledge, and communicative justice*. Duke University Press. https://doi.org/10.1515/9780822374398

Chen, S.-F. [世新大學新聞學系] (2021, May 27). *1 1*陳秀鳳 新冠肺炎疫情下 社群互動平台對記者專業實踐的影響：以中央流行疫情指揮中心直播記者會為例 [11 Chen, Siou-Fong. The impact of social media responses on the professional practices of journalists in the times of COVID-19: Examples from CECC livestreaming news conferences.] [Video]. YouTube. www.youtube.com/watch?v=TOzt15F3CX0

Clayman, S., & Heritage, J. (2002). *The news nnterview: Journalists and public figures on the air*. Cambridge University Press. https://doi.org/10.1017/CBO9780511613623

Dau, D., & Ellis, K. (2023). From Bondi to Fairfield: NSW COVID-19 press conferences, health messaging, and social inequality. *Media International Australia*, *188*(1), 31–51. https://doi.org/10.1177/1329878X221087732

De León, L. (2011). Language socialization and multiparty participation frameworks. In A. Duranti, E. Ochs, & B. B. Schieffelin (Eds.), *The handbook of language socialization* (pp. 81–111). Wiley-Blackwell. https://doi.org/10.1002/9781444342901.ch4

Degani, M. (2022). 'Unite against COVID-19': Jacinda Ardern's discursive approach to the pandemic. In A. Musolff, R. Breeze, K. Kondo, & S. Vilar-Lluch (Eds.), *Pandemic and crisis discourse: Communicating COVID-19 and public health strategy* (pp. 471–486). Bloomsbury Publishing.

Griffiths, J. (2020, April 5). *Taiwan's coronavirus response is among the best globally*. CNN. https://edition.cnn.com/2020/04/04/asia/taiwan-coronavirus-response-who-intl-hnk/index.html

Gumperz, J. J. (1988). *Contextualization and understanding*. Department of Linguistics, University of California at Berkeley. www.degruyter.com/database/COGBIB/entry/cogbib.5061/html

Hyland-Wood, B., Gardner, J., Leask, J., & Ecker, U. K. H. (2021). Toward effective government communication strategies in the era of COVID-19. *Humanities & Social Sciences Communications*, *8*(1), 1–11. https://doi.org/10.1057/s41599-020-00701-w

Jacobs, G. (1999). *Preformulating the news*. John Benjamins. https://doi.org/https://doi.org/10.1075/pbns.60

Jacobs, G. (2011). Press conferences on the Internet: Technology, mediation and access in the news. *Journal of pragmatics*, *43*(7), 1900–1911. https://doi.org/10.1016/j.pragma.2010.09.019

Kalb, M. L. (2018). *Enemy of the people: Trump's war on the press, the new McCarthyism, and the threat to American democracy*. Brookings Institution Press. www.jstor.org/stable/10.7864/j.ctt1zxskqf

Lee, S.-H. (2024a). How pandemic detective narratives potentiate and debilitate trust. *Text & Talk*, *44*(6), 809–841. https://doi.org/10.1515/text-2022-0080

Lee, S.-H. (2024b). Crisis classifications in mobility: Reporting the first COVID death in Taiwan. *Discourse Studies*, *26*(2), 242–261. https://doi.org/10.1177/14614456231219741

Lee, T.-H. (2020, January 22). 武漢肺炎：台灣首例確診者發病後搭機返鄉 台叫停武漢雙向旅遊團 [Wuhan pneumonia: Taiwan's first confirmed case fell ill after returning home by flight; Taiwan suspends two-way travel tours with Wuhan.] BBC News Chinese. www.bbc.com/zhongwen/trad/chinese-news-51202545

Lee, T.-Y. (2021, March 16). 莊人祥被問AZ回嗆「為什麼要告訴你」 引爆網砲轟：所以死了人也不知道？ [Jen-hsiang Chuang was asked about AstraZeneca vaccine and responded sharply, "Why should I tell you?" This sparked waves of online criticism: "So if people die, you wouldn't even know?"]. *China Times*. www.chinatimes.com/realtimenews/20210316001065-260407?chdtv

Lempert, M. (2011). Barack Obama, being sharp: Indexical order in the pragmatics of precision-grip gesture. *Gesture*, *11*(3), 241–270. https://doi.org/10.1075/gest.11.3.01lem

Lu, W.-H. (2020, March 17). 為什麼天天想追「疫情指揮中心記者會」？ [Why do people want to watch "Epidemic Command Center press conference" every day?]. CommonWealth Magazine. https://opinion.cw.com.tw/blog/profile/423/article/9194

Vásquez, C. (2021). Leading with stories: Andrew Cuomo, family narratives and authentic leadership. *Discourse, Context & Media*, *41*, 100507. https://doi.org/10.1016/j.dcm.2021.100507

Wang, C. J., Ng, C. Y., & Brook, R. H. (2020). Response to COVID-19 in Taiwan: Big data analytics, new technology, and proactive testing. *JAMA*, *323*(14), 1341–1342. https://doi.org/10.1001/jama.2020.3151

Wang, S.-F., Lee, H.-C., Chen, H.-Y., & Yang, C.-Y. (2003). SARS 即時定量系統的建立與分析 [Establishment and snalysis of the SARS real-time quantification system]. *Taiwan Epidemiology Bulletin*, *19*(7), 351–365. www.cdc.gov.tw/Uploads/files/201211/0de14273-4dc0-4fc0-aa2e-d1ea9425d44f.pdf

Wei, H.-N., Tai, Y.-S., Ko, H.-Y., & Tsao, K.-L. (2022). 運用新媒體進行 COVID-19 疫情相關衛教及溝通 [Uusing new media for COVID-19 pandemic-related health education and communication]. *Taiwan Epidemiology Bulletin*, *38*(24), 351–365.

Wilkie, C. (2020, May 11). *Trump abruptly ends press conference after reporters challenge him on coronavirus testing*. CNBC. www.cnbc.com/2020/05/11/coronavirus-trump-ends-press-conference-after-reporters-challenge-him-on-testing.html

3 Narrative Classification

During the COVID-19 pandemic, many countries implemented strict border control with the aim of keeping the outbreak at bay or mitigating the spread of new virus variants. Restrictions on human mobility are oftentimes fraught with controversy, particularly when they stipulate who is allowed to enter or leave national territories. The United States shut its southern border to asylum seekers out of fear that the coronavirus would spread in detention facilities and among personnel (Kanno-Youngs & Semple, 2020). China imposed exit bans on citizens' non-essential travel in an effort to enforce its zero-COVID policy (Yeung, 2022). Australia asked international students and visa holders to return to their home countries because Australia needed to prioritize its own citizens (Gibson & Moran, 2020). Such restrictions fortify the boundaries of an imagined community (Anderson, 1983) and the group identities of insider versus outsider, which are often used to rationalize controversial governance.

This chapter argues that restriction communication is prone to controversy when it constructs an identity frame of insider versus outsider to shape public reception of the restriction, especially if there are gaps within and across communicative modes. The example I use to illustrate my argument is the controversy over the Taiwanese government's approach to the children of Chinese and Taiwanese parents during the initial outbreak of the COVID-19 pandemic in early 2020. For clarity, in the remainder of the chapter, "mainland," "Chinese," and "China" are used interchangeably to refer to the People's Republic of China. I use "Taiwan" and "Taiwanese" to refer to the Republic of China[1] (Taiwan).

In response to the initial outbreak in China in February 2020, the Taiwanese government barred Chinese visitors from entering Taiwan, including the children of Chinese and Taiwanese couples because these children were not Taiwanese citizens and might hold Chinese citizenship. Having further considered the children of Chinese and Taiwanese couples, the Mainland Affairs Council in Taiwan subsequently revised the restriction to allow the children to enter Taiwan. However, the revised restriction sparked criticism from the media and the public due to a lack of understanding about this marginalized group of individuals, the fear of the COVID-19 outbreak in

DOI: 10.4324/9781003545002-3

China, and the enduring struggle between China and Taiwan over the sovereignty of Taiwan. The revised restriction thus amplified all sensitive tensions about nationality, pandemic origin, and sovereignty.

Confronted with this criticism, the minister of the Mainland Affairs Council revised the restriction a second time by allowing the children entry only under special conditions: if they were under 18 years old and had no relative in China who could take care of them. In announcing these changes, the minister strove to clarify the changes and the children's challenging circumstances. This endeavor was reflected in the minister's use of narratives and categories that gave life and breath to the pandemic identity of the minor children. However, the minister's communication failed to convince the media and the public, instead sparking even more criticism and confusion. Eventually, the government revoked the changes and banned all Chinese citizens from entering Taiwan, including the children of Chinese and Taiwanese couples who were not Taiwanese citizens. This chapter investigates why the minister's narration and classification failed to create public acceptance and support.

Ideally, a combination of narration and classification is powerful enough to make information accessible to the public, especially when both communicative modes exemplify the two modes of thought—paradigmatic and narrative—that Bruner (1987) suggests individuals rely on to organize their lived experiences and interpret the world. This chapter takes a different point of departure by investigating the type of narrative and paradigmatic relationships that spark public resistance and criticism. In the analyzed case, the gaps within and between each communicative mode propel the social identification of the children as outsiders and increase public distrust of the minister. My aim in researching this unsuccessful interplay is not simply to point out the pitfalls. Instead, I seek to uncover the challenges of integrating paradigmatic and narrative talk into a coherent and cohesive whole. A better understanding of these challenges would help scholars and practitioners (re)envisage restriction communication as a synergy of various communicative modes rather than a list of do's and don'ts in public-health-communication documents.

In what follows, I first introduce Bruner's (1987) constructs of paradigmatic and narrative thinking and discuss how they are operationalized in this chapter to explore the controversial episode. I then provide background information to contextualize the episode, along with an overview of the data used to understand the episode. Subsequently, I present my multimodal analysis of the minister's speech. The analysis underscores the multimodal features that led to the public reception of the children as outsiders. Finally, I summarize the key findings and deduce implications.

Two Modes of Thinking and Talk: Paradigmatic vs. Narrative

Bruner (1987) argued that there exist at least two modes of thought that individuals rely upon to construe the world and organize their lived experiences: paradigmatic and narrative. To think paradigmatically is to search for truth through procedures such as verification, falsification, generalization, and categorization. These procedures align with the call for depoliticizing COVID-19 communication through science-based communication that foregrounds the search for universal truth and objective fact in logico-scientific evidence (Chan et al., 2023). To think narratively is to put narrative's "timeless miracles into the particulars of experience, and to locate that experience in time and place" (Bruner, 1987, p. 13). Narrative thinking also imbues experiences with meaning, and successful narration grants audiences access to the lives and minds of characters, thereby making narratives "magnets for empathy" (Bruner, 1986, p. 21). Additionally, narratives help set the parameters of appropriate response to a perceived threat (Garro & Mattingly, 2001).

As these definitions suggest, a logical argument and a vivid story are essentially different. Their differences are further reflected in the worlds they construct. Paradigmatic reasoning engenders theories, principles, and criteria that can stand up to the test of empirical proof. Narrative reasoning creates not only a story world that entails characters, actions, goals, settings, and means, but also a psychic reality that underscores the subjectivity of the characters, including their thoughts and feelings.

Another defining difference is their conceptualization of causality. Paradigmatic causality is a search for universal truth conditions as in "if X, then Y," whereas narrative causality links two events as in "The king died, and then the queen died" (Bruner, 1987, p. 12). Put simply, verification, falsification, generalization, and categorization characterize paradigmatic reasoning, whereas the intersection of plight, character, and consciousness is the hallmark of narrative reasoning.

Despite their differences, both modes often live side by side. Ochs et al. (1992) observed that at the dinner table of the middle-class US family, as children learn to co-narrate their life experiences, they also engage in the problem-solving, theory-building, and perspective-taking that underlie logico-scientific thought and discourse. In a language classroom, paradigmatic and narrative talk combine to help an instructor fulfill institutional mandates while nurturing students' interests (Lee, 2020). Even in science class, narratives foster learning by enacting teaching in previous classes (Andrée et al., 2017) or interweaving personal experiences with general scientific principles (Peterson, 2009). Furthermore, many scientific theories and hypotheses start as stories and gradually reach maturity as empirical discoveries. Wald (2008) argued that epidemiology was "at once to read and to write the epidemic as a story of detection with predictive value" (p. 23).

Both modes of thinking and talk are thus indispensable to each other. The absence of, or overreliance on, either is detrimental to fully understanding the world, particularly when it comes to matters of life or death in public health. In perilous times, the separation of paradigmatic and narrative communication thwarts efforts to correctly and quickly diagnose an epidemic. Consider Briggs and Mantini-Briggs's (2016) ethnographic study of a mysterious epidemic in the rainforest of eastern Venezuela in 2008. Health officials devalued indigenous parents' narratives about their diseased children because the parents had no medical training. Instead, epidemiologists presented their images of powerful medical and political figures by strategically juxtaposing medical terminology, colloquial expressions, and terms used only within healthcare institutions.

Effective crisis communication about restrictions requires the skillful integration of both modes of thought and talk to contextualize general categories and to ground the communication in facts. If restriction communication relies exclusively on narratives, the communication is personal and particular, not generalizable, thus making it difficult to engender public cooperation. Likewise, without narratives, restriction communication may become abstract and detached from reality, rendering it difficult to disseminate information across social groups.

Paradigmatic Classifications and Narrative Chronotopes

Building on this wealth of literature about paradigmatic and narrative interplay, I analyze the Taiwanese minister's speech that attempted the successful interplay but ultimately sparked controversy. Paradigmatic thinking is operationalized in my analysis as classifications by which "categories are established, instantiated, idealized, and related one to the other to form a system" (Bruner, 1987, p. 12). This system was referenced by officials to facilitate their description and explanation of COVID-related measures, such as who was permitted to travel under the restrictions. Central to the process of paradigmatic classification is an understanding of what something is equivalent to ("categorization") or different from ("particularization"), to quote Billig (1985). That is, categorization involves sorting an instance into a general category or grouping with similar instances, whereas particularization removes an instance from a general category or other instances because the instance is considered different and thus unfit. In essence, to classify is to sort by correspondence and difference. Furthermore, like other discursive practices associated with paradigmatic reasoning, paradigmatic classification requires that language use be overt and explicit, never inconsistent or contradictory.

For the purpose of this study, narrative is both a speech genre and a social practice that constructs social identity and imbues life experiences with meaning (De Fina & Georgakopoulou, 2011). On this basis, I focus on how identity work—e.g., behaviors, discourses, and interactional patterns—is organized or referenced within specific time-space configurations or chronotopes (Bakhtin, 1981; Blommaert & De Fina, 2017). For instance, in the narrative I analyze, I show how the children's identities were constructed and enacted in specific times (past, present, future) and places (China and Taiwan) that constitute various layers of chronotopes (e.g., remote-past birth in China vs. recent-past education in Taiwan). In his attempt to convince the public of the revised restriction in the here-and-now of the narrating event, the minister foregrounded certain chronotopes that highlight the ingroup identity of

Table 3.1 The analytical framework of narrative classification

Paradigmatic classifications	Categorization: an instance is grouped into a category Particularization: an instance is extracted from a category
Narrative chronotopes	Time: past, present, or future Space: China or Taiwan

Taiwanese and backgrounded others associated with the outgroup identity of Chinese. Chronotopic comparison, juxtaposition, or lamination, which is called cross-chronotopic alignment (Koven, 2019), is one of the foci of my analysis.

One goal of the current study is to explore the multimodal interplay between narrative chronotopes and paradigmatic classifications in communicating restrictions. A better understanding of the interplay would help officials reconceptualize restriction communication not as compartmentalized rules for stipulating the do's and don'ts, but as a nexus of different modes of discourses that construct group identities to mediate the public reception of restrictions. Table 3.1 presents the analytical framework adopted in this chapter to understand the interface of paradigmatic and narrative thinking as well as their analytical focus. In the remainder of the chapter, I will draw on the framework to analyze the minister's speech and answer the following questions: What identities does the minister construct through narrative chronotopes and paradigmatic classifications? Why do the minister's narration and classification fail to persuade the audiences online (i.e., online viewers) and offline (i.e., journalists at conferences)?

Context

Taiwanese Ingroup and Chinese Outgroup

Given the tensions between China and Taiwan over Taiwan's sovereignty, the issue of citizenship for Chinese spouses and their underage children is a delicate one. At the core of the issue is national allegiance. In a more balanced news report, Tsao and Guo (2020) explored different challenges faced by Chinese-Taiwanese couples during the COVID-19 pandemic. Their report draws on perspectives from law, sociology, public health, and cross-Taiwan-Strait relations, revealing that while opinions varied regarding how the government should address the issue, Taiwanese immigration policies and border restriction orders reflected societal distrust and aversion toward China.

For example, before the COVID-19 pandemic, it had been more complex and required more effort for Chinese spouses to obtain Taiwanese citizenship compared to spouses of other foreign nationalities. The pandemic, along with border restrictions, only exacerbated the situation. When Taiwan announced a ban on Chinese spouses and their children without Taiwanese citizenship from entering the country on February 11, 2020, foreign nationals were still permitted to enter Taiwan even if they had traveled through China to Taiwan (Bureau of Consular Affairs, 2020). Moreover, when many countries closed their borders to foreign nationals in 2020 to control the COVID-19 outbreak, the Central Epidemic Command Center (CECC) emphasized 'nationals first' when determining who had the priority of entering Taiwan (Huang, 2020). The 'nationals first' principle excluded Chinese spouses and their children from being recognized as Taiwanese nationals if they only held a residency visa through marriage to a Taiwanese citizen. Tsai (2023) argued that the exclusion reflects the government's broader political drive to distinguish "Taiwanese" from "Chinese" as both a national and ethnic identity.

Additionally, distrust toward China deepened in Taiwanese society after new COVID-19 cases were detected following the return of Taiwanese businesspeople from China, as well as in the first charter flight between China and Taiwan. Due to these incidents, an official from the Mainland Affairs Council noted that the government had to revoke the relaxation of border controls on Chinese spouses and their underage children because there was 'insufficient support from the society' (Tsao & Guo, 2020). Chinese spouses and their children were not allowed to enter Taiwan until later in 2020 (Taiwan Centers for Disease Control, 2020). These incidents highlight a dominant ideology prevailing in Taiwanese society throughout 2020: Taiwanese ingroup versus Chinese outgroup. Families of Chinese-Taiwanese couples were thrust into the position of confronting the ideological divide.

Timeline of Restriction Changes

This chapter focuses on the episode about the travel ban and minor children because it became highly contentious online. Public online discourses strongly opposed the relaxation of border controls for these children, which ultimately forced government officials to revoke the policy (Huang, 2020). The episode also influenced public perceptions of social minorities, whose identities were suddenly subject to scrutiny and even criticism. The language used in the episode was mediatized through live-streams and TV news, shaping public discussions around the children of Chinese-Taiwanese couples.

I identified three recordings and a media release that together contain all sequences about the changes to the mobility restriction for the children. Table 3.2 presents the timeline of the changes across the recordings and a media release. Table 3.2 shows that over time, the entry conditions became increasingly strict and eventually resulted in a ban on the children's entry. Furthermore, the status of the officials announcing the stricter restrictions grew from a director, to a minister, to a council, and finally to a commander, reflecting growing public backlash against the changes and the government's attempt to assuage the backlash.

The Minister's Announcement

My analysis focuses on the minister of the Mainland Affairs Council's announcement regarding changes to border restrictions, along with live-chat

Table 3.2 Timeline of restriction changes

Date and time	*Announcer*	*Who can enter Taiwan*
February 11, 2020, 2:00 pm	Director of the Mainland Affairs Council	Compatriots or Chinese spouses' Chinese children with the visa of the special case of permanent residency or the permanent residence for visiting family or relatives
February 11, 2020, 7:00 pm	Minister of the Mainland Affairs Council	The minor children of Chinese and Taiwanese couples. The children do not have relatives in China who are able to take care of them.
February 11, 2020, media release published after conference	The Mainland Affairs Council	The minor children of Chinese and Taiwanese couples. The children do not have relatives in China who are able to take care of them. Both parents are in Taiwan.
February 12, 2020, 1:00 pm	Commander of the Central Epidemic Command Center	Chinese spouses' children cannot enter Taiwan if they are not Taiwanese nationals.

comments that accompanied the YouTube live-stream of his speech. I chose the minister's announcement because it provoked the most intense public controversy and sharp criticism, ultimately forcing the CECC commander to revoke the changes one day after the announcement.

The announcement was delivered at an impromptu press conference in the evening, five hours after the initial border relaxation policies were introduced to the public. Due to the impromptu nature of the conference, only two CECC officials co-presented with the minister, as opposed to the full panel typically present during the daily COVID-19 press conference. Figure 3.1 shows the setting of the press conference when the minister announced the change.

My following analysis seeks to understand why the attempt to promote acceptance and support instead yielded strong public confusion and disapproval. To do so, I analyze the multimodalities of the minister's narrative and paradigmatic discourses and triangulate the multimodal analysis with online viewers' comments in live chat responses and journalists' questions during the question-and-answer time. This derives a more nuanced view of the communicative problems in the speech.

Analysis

This section presents my multimodal analysis of the minister's speech. I segmented the speech into four excerpts. Each excerpt underscores pandemic identities that (dis)align with Taiwan through the minister's use of multimodal resources. I triangulated the analysis with online viewers'

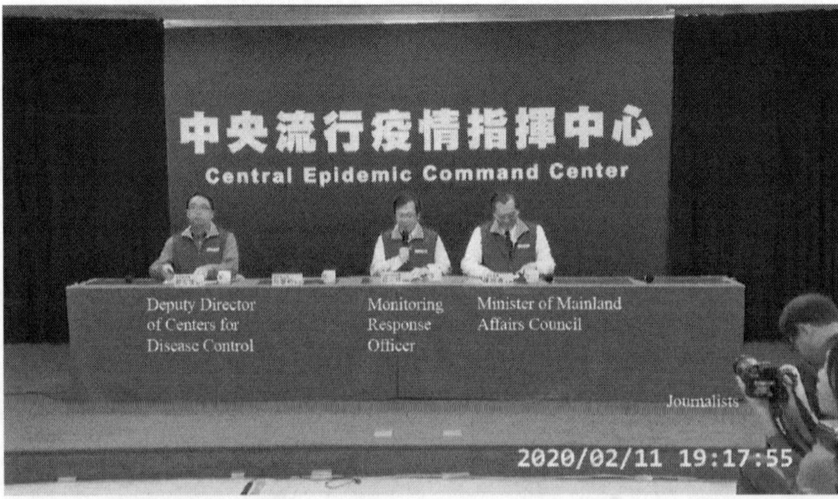

Figure 3.1 The impromptu conference for announcing the revision of border relaxation.

Source: Taiwan Centers for Disease Control, February 11, 2020. www.youtube.com/watch?v=cBdPsHpOkG4

comments and journalists' questions to pinpoint the communicative problems that might have led to public confusion and criticism.

Particularizing Chinese Spouses' Chinese Relatives

Soon after the conference began, the minister of the Mainland Affairs Council updated the public about the changes in mobility restrictions. In Excerpt 1, he explicitly stated that the purpose of his speech was to clarify the mobility restriction policy that had been announced earlier that day.

Excerpt 1

1	Minister	<F啊F>各位媒體呃=小姐先生, ..呃大家晚安 ..大家好啊.	Ah media representatives. Uh ladies and gentlemen. Uh good evening everyone. How's everyone?
2		..不好意思.	Excuse me.

3	...呃因為我們下午..有宣布了一些(THROAT)<MRC管制措施MRC>的政策齁, ...(.7)那= ..可能在用詞上<P啊P>不是=很清楚, ..所以我在這個機會啊..來特別來說明齁.	Uh because this afternoon we announced some (border) control measures hm. Hm, maybe (our) language was not very clear. So I am taking this opportunity to specifically explain (it) hm.
4	...那絕對不是<F外面F>所說的, ..呃= 開放=這個=陸配的大陸親人..來探親齁.	Hm it is absolutely not what has been said outside (the conference). Uh (that) mainland spouses' mainland relatives (are) allowed to come to visit family, OK.
5	...絕對不是這個東西齁.	(It is) absolutely not this kind of thing, OK.
6	...那=, ..這個起心-這個政策, ..呃起心動念-,我先來講一個故事.	Hm the moti- this policy, uh the motive (behind this policy). Let me first tell a story.
7	讓大家瞭解說我們這個政策到底想幹什麼齁.	To help everyone understand what exactly our- this policy is trying to do.

As Excerpt 1 shows, in a metadiscursive statement, the minister framed the source of the controversy as a misunderstanding and stated the purpose of his speech (3). The metadiscourse attributed the controversy to a language problem, not a problem with the policy itself. He then drew on particularization (Billig, 1985) to position Chinese spouses' Chinese relatives as outsiders and exclude them from the category of individuals who could benefit from the revised restriction (4). The extreme case formulation (Pomerantz, 1986) 絕對 'absolutely' was repeated to strengthen the particularization (4–5). In an abrupt move, the minister prefaced an upcoming narration (6) with the goal of helping the public understand the motive behind the change (7).

The abruptness of the minister's remarks was noticed and challenged by several online commenters, with responses such as 'Telling a story?' and 'I don't want to hear stories.' Most commenters rejected the minister's framing of the issue as a miscommunication, asserting instead that 'The Mainland Affairs Council can't figure out the problem.' They interpreted the minister's metadiscursive statement as an attempt to advocate for the relaxation policy: 'Force it' or 'Still try to make excuses.'

Narrating Xiao Ming

The minister then drew on narrative to chronotopically construct an identity aligned more closely with Taiwan than with China. The narrative in Excerpt 2 centered on the odyssey undertaken by a fictional character, 小明 Xiao Ming.

The pseudonym Xiao Ming signalled familiarity and closeness as the prefix 小 'Xiao' literally means little and can be used to address friends who are the same age or younger than oneself.

Excerpt 2

1	Minister	...<F<HI這個國人啊HI>F>, ...呃=在大陸, ..啊不管是經商啦<A或什麼什麼X A>, ..啊就=, ..在大陸呢, ...娶了大陸的配偶, ...(.7)那麼生了=一個小孩子.	Uh a compatriot, uh on the mainland. Uh whether (he was there) for business or whatever whatever. Uh then on the mainland (he) married a mainland spouse and then has a child.
2		..<P啊P>假設是小明.	Ah suppose (the child is called) Xiao Ming.
3		..<P齁小明P>.	OK, Xiao Ming.
4		...(.7)<F那麼=F>在大陸<P呃=P>一段時間之後呢, ...那=, ..舉家呢, ...就回到台灣來.	So uh, after a period of time on the mainland, then, the entire family moved back to Taiwan.

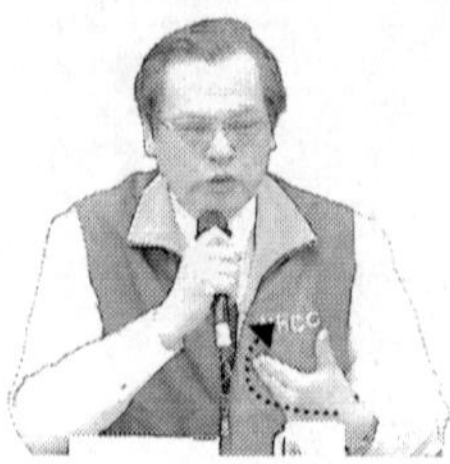

5		...(.9)<A那就X回到台灣來A>.	Then moved back to Taiwan.
6		...(.8)<F<HI那麼HI>F>, ...這個小明呢, ..因為=他在台灣呢他沒有戶籍.	So uh, Xiao Ming. Because he[2] has no household registration in Taiwan.
7		...<P齁他沒有戶籍P>.	Hm he has no household registration.
8		<F爸爸F>雖然是我們中華民國的國民, ...齁, ..可是他..在=..大陸出生.	Although (his) father is (one of) our compatriots of the Republic of China[1]. OK. But he (Xiao Ming) was born on the mainland.

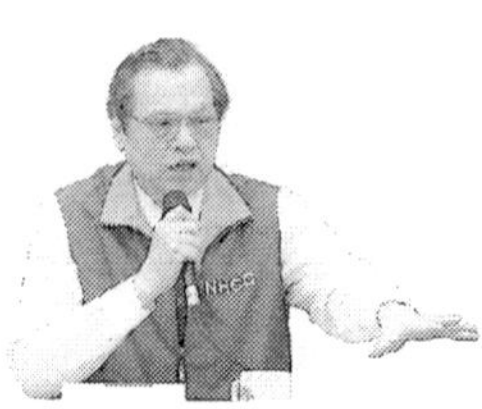

9	齁在大陸出生.	Hm born on the mainland.
10	...所以呢..他跟著爸爸媽媽回到台灣來=.	So he came back to Taiwan with his parents.

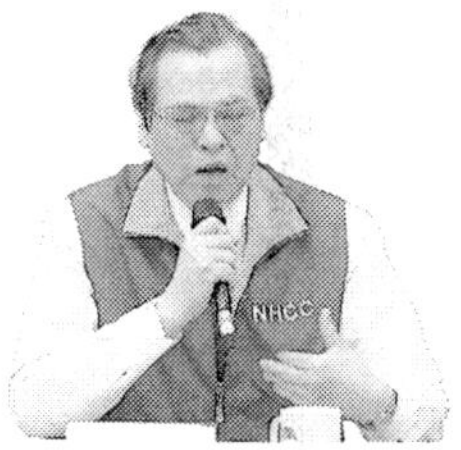

11	...他是以一個..<MRC長期= MRC>..啊這個=, ...<MRC專案啊蛤= MRC>,這個=..<P呃P>, ...<F這個專案長期居留F>或者長期的探親呃這個居留的方式在台灣..呃生活.	He .. uh lives in Taiwan through a .. permanent-.. uh this .. special case uh hm this .. uh ... the special case of permanent residency (visa) or the permanent residence (visa) for visiting family or relatives.
12	..<P齁P>.	OK.
13	..那這個生活<RH呃一段的時間=, ..也在這邊上小學, ...啊拿了健保..<P啊P>RH>, ...<A其實他在台灣已經很久<P的一段時間了啦P>A>.	Uh hm (he) lives (in Taiwan) uh for a period of time. (He) also goes to an elementary school here (and) uh obtains (national) health insurance .. uh. Actually, he has been in Taiwan for a very long period of time.
14	...(.9)<F然後呢F>, ..過年了..就跟著<F媽媽F>,可能回到媽媽的<F娘家F>.	And then, when Lunar New Year comes, (he) follows (his) mother to maybe go back to (his) mother's family home.
15	...到大陸去看<TW阿公阿嬤TW>.	To visit (his) grandparents on the mainland.
16	..齁.	OK.
17	...(1.2) <F<HI那他因為沒有中華民國的身分HI>F>, ...所以現在因為為了<MRC防疫MRC>, ..<F大陸人士F>就不能進來.	Uh because he has no identity status of the Republic of China. So because of Covid preventative measures, mainlanders can't enter (Taiwan).

18	...啊大陸人士就不能進來.	Ah mainlanders can't enter (Taiwan).
19	...結果..<HI這個小孩子HI>, ..<A小明這個小孩子A>,其實..本來長期在台灣..生活很久了.	As a result, this child. Xiao Ming, this child. In fact, (he) has been living in Taiwan for a very long period of time.
20	..<RH也念了小學了, ..念了中學了, 拿了健保的RH>.	(He) also studied at an elementary school, studied at a high school, and has national insurance.
21	...但<F<HI因為HI>F>, ...(1.2)這樣的一個..防疫的措施以後, ...他沒有辦法回來.	But because this kind .. of Covid-preventive measures, he can't come back.

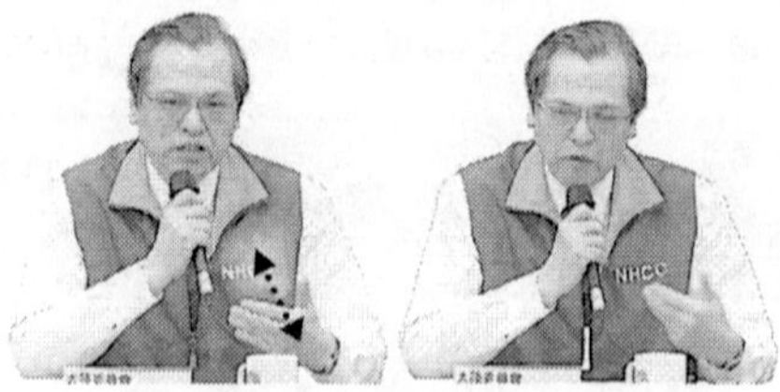

In Excerpt 2, the minister developed the character of Xiao Ming by describing his multiple trips between China and Taiwan. The narration of the trips conjured for viewers a sense of Xiao Ming's affinity with Taiwan. The affinity became evident in the space-time contrast between China and Taiwan, which was anchored in the storytelling world. Specifically, Xiao Ming's tie with Taiwan was created through the motion verbs of 來 'come' (toward the narrator) and 去 'go' (away from the narrator) that helped the audiences conceptualize the direction in which Xiao Ming was traveling. That is, the migration to Taiwan was toward the narrator (the minister) in the storytelling world, as shown in the frequent use of 來 'come' (4, 5, 10, 17, 18, 21), whereas the trip to visit grandparents in China during the Lunar New Year holiday was away from the narrator (the minister), as indicated by the motion verb 去 'go' (15), which was used only once.

Imagistically, the minister embodied the proxemics to Taiwan in his gestures. Moving to Taiwan was shown by a cupped-hand gesture directed toward the minister's central body (4, 10, 21). Born in China was spatialized by the gesture of an open hand, palm prone, that was peripheral to the minister's body (8). The barriers to Xiao Ming's return to Taiwan were presented in the metaphoric gesture of an open hand, palm facing the minister, that moved back and forth to block the passage toward the minister's central body (21). In addition to space, the chronotopic contrast between Taiwan and China materialized in the degree adverb 很 'very' and the adjective久 'long' that modified the length of time in Taiwan (19, 13) and the absence of these modifiers from the description of the time in China (4).

Discursively, the repetition of time-space configurations (13, 19–20) revealed the minister's attempt to emphasize Xiao Ming's sameness to other Taiwanese children who attended school and participated in the national health insurance system even though the repetition disrupted the linear progressivity of the telling—i.e., born in China → migrated to Taiwan → visited grandparents in China → cannot return to Taiwan. This constellation of multimodal resources foregrounds the minister's attempt to render the affected children's close relationship with Taiwan recognizable. The affinity legitimizes the revised restriction.

Despite his efforts, in his explanation the minister captured only the rights (i.e., school education and national health insurance) Xiao Ming had engaged but not his obligations, echoing the dominant discourse that cross-Strait returnees exploit social welfare in Taiwan but do not recognize Taiwan's sovereignty (Lin & Chung, 2016). As a result, the minister's instantiation and reiteration of Xiao Ming affinity with Taiwan (13, 19–20) reinforced the social differentiation of Xiao Ming as an outsider (Yang, 2021). Some of the online comments also underscored the children's differences rather than sameness: 'just want Chinese citizenship and also want Taiwan's (national) health insurance'; and 'Not getting Taiwanese citizenship. Then it's taking advantage of the (national) health insurance!' Other commenters more directly classified the children as outgroups, either in general ('He is not Taiwanese. None of my business.') or specifically as part of the Chinese outgroup ('A Chinese citizen. China will take good care of him. Don't worry'). The narrative of Xiao Ming failed to prompt any online comment that identified the children as part of the Taiwanese ingroup.

Categorizing the Minor Children in China

Following the narration, in Excerpt 3, the minister elaborated on the reason behind the officials' decision to review and revise the restriction, allowing the children to enter Taiwan. He introduced criteria for classifying who would be permitted entry under the new restriction regulations.

Excerpt 3

1	Minister	…(1.0)那=, …這個事情, … (.8)呃=在=因為我們..這個, ..為了防疫的<F需要F>, ..那..讓這個=… 大陸人士啊, ..呃..這個..停-停止呃盡可能停止交流..齁.	Hm, this matter- uh in- because we- this- for the sake of Covid prevention, hm let the- ah uh this- stop- stop uh- try to stop social contact with mainlanders. OK.

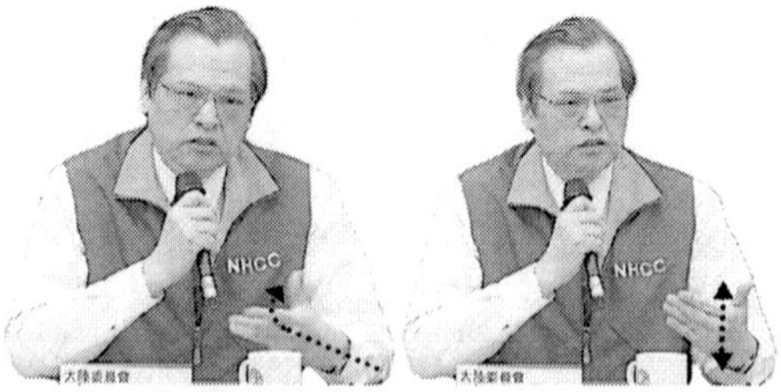

2	..那=..這一塊的人..他因為沒有中華民國國籍, ...他<F回不來啊F>.	Hm, this group of people. They do not have nationality of the Republic of China. They can't come back.

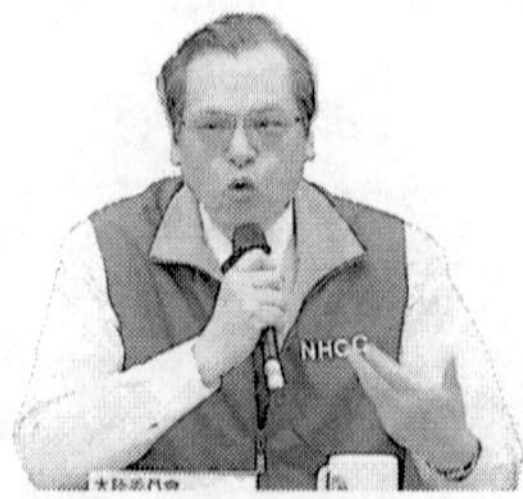

3	...<A他其實XA>他是回不來啊.	They actually- they can't come back.

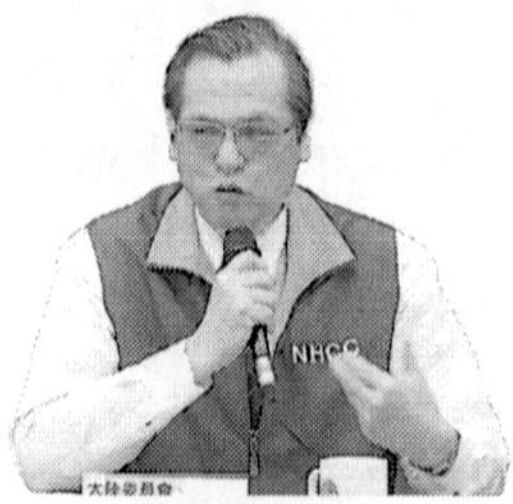

4	..那這個事情啊, ..<P唉=P>, ...(.8)陳情了很久了啊, ..已經有一個禮拜多了.	Hm, this matter, uh, (they) have been petitioning for a long time. It has been more than a week.
5	..<P齁一個禮拜多了..齁P>.	Hm, more than a week, OK.
6	...所以=呃我們政策上, ...(.7)那對於這個<A他本來就在台灣生活的小孩=A>, ...因為過年, ...回去媽媽的娘家看, ...(.7)外公外婆, ...然後現在回不來.	So uh in our policy, for the children who have lived in Taiwan and went back to (their) mothers' family home to visit grandparents because of Chinese New Year, and then can't come back now.

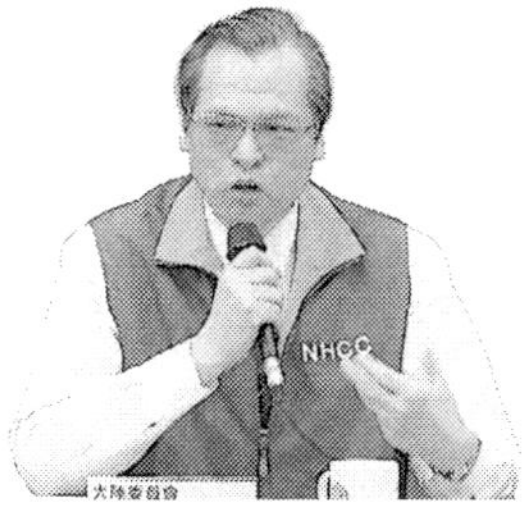

7	..所以我們做一個...人道的考量, ...啊讓他能夠<P回來P>.	So we made a humanitarian consideration to let them come back.

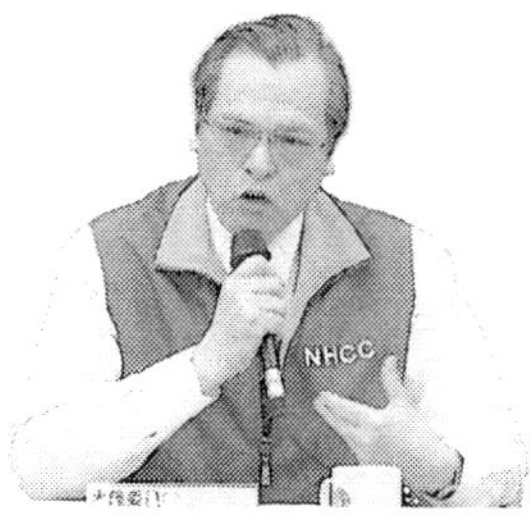

8	<A哦其實就是讓他回來A>.	Uh, to actually let them come back.
9	...<F<HI不過HI>F>, ..呃<A因為社會反應A>..很-這個=..<A有各方面的<F意見F>A>.	But uh because the public reacted very- this- there are all kinds of opinions
10	...(.7)再加上現在防疫啊..重於一切.	Plus now Covid prevention is prioritized over anything else.
11	..齁.	OK.
12	..所以=..我們這個政策..有所調整.	So our- this policy has some adjustments.
13	..<A齁我們這個政策有調整齁A>.	Uh, we- this policy has adjustments
14	...<F也就是說F>, ...(.7)這些小孩子, ...(.7)<F第一個F>, ...如果他是未成年=?, ...<F第二個F>, ...他在大陸沒有親人來照顧他, ...(.8)齁, ...(1.0)第一個他未成年.	That is, these children, first is if they are underage. Second, they have no relative to take care of them on the mainland. OK. The first is they are underage.
15	..第二他在大陸沒有親人.	The second is they have no relative on the mainland.

16	..<P齁P>.	OK.
17	..<TW阿公阿嬤TW><A或者沒有親人有能力來照顧他A>.	Grandparents or no (other) relative who have the ability to take care of them.
18	...(.9)這個時候, ...X他必須專案, ...來提出申請.	In this situation, they have to apply for a special case (consideration).
19	...啊我們...考量各種<F意見F>, ...<P啊P>, ..專案來-來-si-..呃審查.	Ah we will consider all kinds of opinions. Ah (we will) review it uh as as a si- special case.
20	...<P齁P>.	OK.
21	..再...給予以准駁<P齁P>.	Then (we will) make a decision hm.

In Excerpt 3, while the minister continued to underscore Xiao Ming's connection to Taiwan through the return gesture (1, 2, 3, 6, 7), barrier gesture (1), and motion verbs (2, 3, 6, 7, 8), he gradually withdrew from narrative reasoning and stepped into the paradigmatic mode. The minister signaled the modal transition by abandoning the address term of Xiao Ming in the narrative and adopting the noun phrases of 這一塊的人 'this group of people' (2) and 這些小孩 'these children' (14) to refer to the children who were in limbo due to the restriction. While the third-person singular pronoun 他 'he' remained in use, the pronoun was used to refer to the established identity of this group of individuals instead of Xiao Ming himself because Chinese noun phrases are flexibly specified if they can be understood from context (Li & Thompson, 1981).

Additionally, according to the narrative (Excerpt 2), Xiao Ming had no household registration in Taiwan, was born in China, and was not a citizen of Taiwan; however, the paradigmatic talk (Excerpt 3) explicitly indicated that these individuals had no Taiwanese nationality and thus could not return to Taiwan (2). This contrast underscores the paradigmatic mode's proclivity for overt meaning.

Finally, a defining feature of paradigmatic talk appears in the use of the metalanguage of 第一 'first' and 第二 'second' (14–15) to introduce the juridical time of 未成年 'underage' and disconnect the children from China: 他在大陸沒有親人來照顧他 'no relatives to take care of them on the mainland.' The two criteria not only redefined the identity of the individuals who could enter Taiwan under the revised restriction but also reinforced the bond individuals form with Taiwan by severing ties with China. This transition from narrative to paradigmatic discourse moves beyond the specific to derive a more generalizable, categorical system.

However, a problem appeared when the classification (Excerpt 3) and narration (Excerpt 2) were in juxtaposition. That is, the stipulation of the second criterion, i.e., the absence of a relative in China who could attend to the children (Excerpt 3, lines 14 and 17), contradicted the prior narrative that Xiao Ming had traveled to China with his mother (Excerpt 2, line 14) who would have been able to take care of him there. This explains why later during the question-and-answer time, a reporter bafflingly asked 爸媽回來了，把小明留在那? '[His] parents came back and left Xiao Ming there?'

The minister's intonation further complicated the situation. That is, though the minister repeated the criteria for the classification to underscore the restriction change (Excerpt 3, 14–15), his intonation unit in line 15 was a standalone complete intonation. This prosodic feature along with the subsequent discourse marker 齁 'OK' (16) led to the interpretation of a journalist and several online viewers that the minister was contradicting himself: in the narrative, Xiao Ming was visiting his grandparents in China, but the classification required children to have 在大陸沒有親人 'no relative on the mainland.' The misunderstanding was epitomized in a reporter's question asked later during the question and answer time, 這個你不就自相矛盾了嗎？ 'Isn't that a contradiction of yourself?' and an online viewer's recontextualization, 'No relatives (on the mainland). How could the children go to the mainland to visit relatives?'

Finally, paradigmatic reasoning emphasizes the procedures for verification, falsification, and categorization (Bruner 1987). It was challenging, if not impossible, to verify or falsify whether the minor children had relatives in China to take care of them, as a reporter also commented when the floor was opened for taking questions from journalists: 你要怎麼-怎麼確定說他沒有辦法這-這邊真的是沒有親人可以照顧，沒有能力撫養? 'How do you determine that they have no way – that there is really no way at all to take care of and no ability to support (the children)?'

The incompleteness and contradiction in the official accounts failed to support the classification of the children as Taiwanese. Instead, they reinforced some online viewers' perception of the children and their mothers as part of the Chinese outgroup. Comments such as '(they) are just Chinese. So much nonsense' and 'A Chinese Xiao Ming destroys the whole of Taiwan' exemplify this sentiment.

Categorizing Our Children and Particularizing Chinese Spouses' Chinese Relatives

Excerpt 4 presents the final sequence of the speech, in which the minister stressed the rationale behind revising the restriction and reiterated the entry criteria.

Excerpt 4

1	Minister	...<F當然這個會隨著疫情的F>..這個發展, ..而所調整.	Of course this will be adjusted according to the development of the pandemic.
2		..<P齁而所調整.	Hm, (it) will be adjusted.

3	...齁P>.	OK.
4	...所以..以上簡單跟大家說明.	So that's all (I want) to explain to everyone.
5	齁<F<HI絕對不是開放HI>陸配的大陸親人<A來探親F>, 沒有沒有這回事A>.	Hm, it is absolutely not about allowing mainland spouses' mainland relatives to come to visit family. No, that's not true.

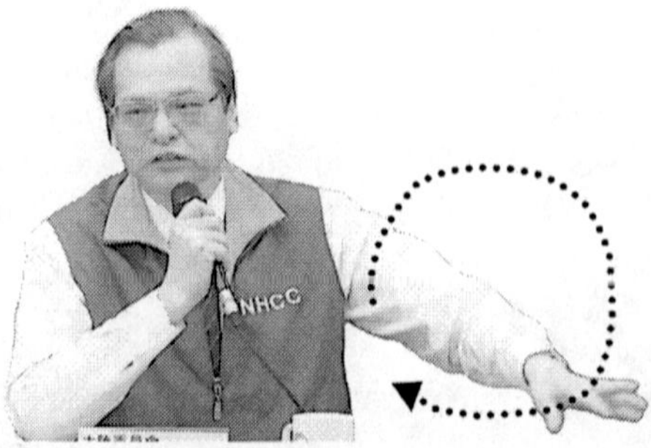

6	齁.	OK.
7	是<F原來我們在這裡F>生活的小孩..讓他回來啊.	It's about letting our children who originally live here to come back.

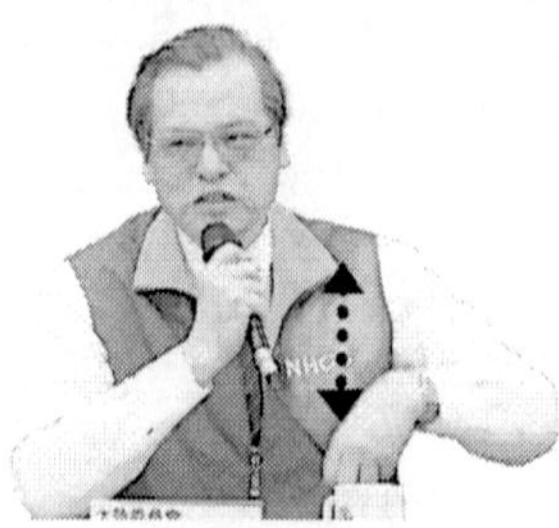

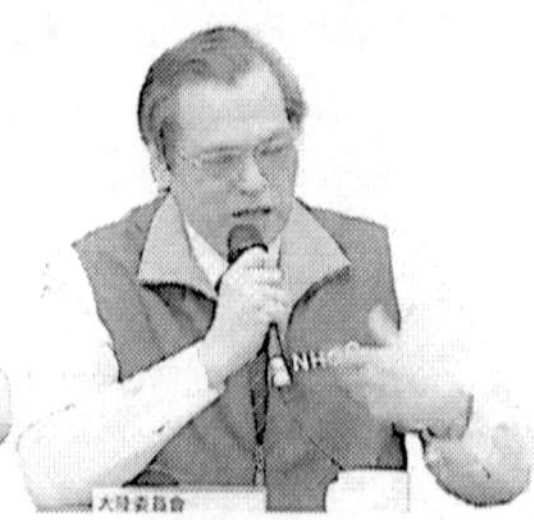

8	..<P讓他回來P>.	To let them come back.

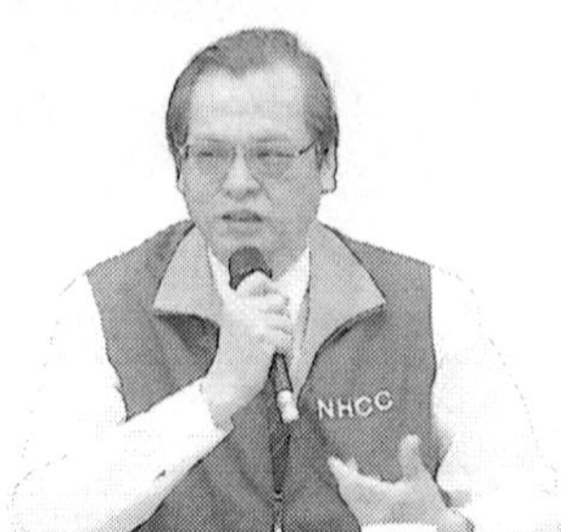

9	..<A但是因為為了疫情上的一個<F管控需要A>, ..現在F>.. 啊我們調整, ..<F除非F>, ..<A第一個他是未成年A>.	But due to the need to control the pandemic, now, ah we make adjustments. (They can't enter Taiwan) unless first, they are underage.
10	..<A<F除非他大陸沒有親人能夠照顧他F>A>.	Unless they have no relatives to take care of them on the mainland.
11	..夠.	OK.
12	..你不能讓他流浪街頭嘛.	You can't let them become homeless.
13	..這個時候, 你專案提出申請, ..我們專案來審查各種意見..在予以准駁.	In such cases, you apply for a special case (consideration). We will review it as a special case by considering all kinds of opinions and then approve or reject it accordingly.
14	..<A以上A>.	This concludes (my report).

As Excerpt 4 shows, the minister contrasted the there-and-then of China and the here-and-now of Taiwan to reiterate who could or could not enter Taiwan. He reiterated the children's alignment with Taiwan and disalignment with China through the construction 不是 … 是 'it's not … it is…' (5–8). The construction brought to the forefront the discursive practices of particularization and categorization. Unlike the particularization seen at the beginning of his speech (Excerpt 1), the particularization of the there-and-then of China was emphasized this time not just verbally—through the extreme case formulation 絕對 'absolutely'—but also, and more importantly, multimodally—with an open hand drawing circles away from the central body (5). In contrast, the categorization created a sense of intimacy through the use of a term of endearment, the first-person plural pronoun 我們 'our,' as well as the spatial deictic 在這裡 'here' and the motion verb 回來 'come back' (7). The term of endearment and deictic overlapped with the deictic beating gesture of a fisted hand moving up and down to underscore the here-and-now of Taiwan.

Subsequently, the minister reiterated the official classification of minor children through the metadiscourse operator 第一個 'first' and the linking adverb 除非 'unless' in parallel (9–10). To further justify the decision, the minister used the indefinite second-person pronoun 你 'you' to engage the online and offline audiences in a hypothetical moral frame in which the children would have become homeless (12) had there been no change to the restriction.

Similar to the end of Excerpt 3, the end of Excerpt 4 shows how the minister drew on multiple linguistic features to reiterate hierarchical power and objective rationality: the institutional deictic 我們 'we' (13), the extreme case formulation 各種意見 'all kinds of' (13), and the official register 予以准駁

'approve or reject it accordingly' (13) and 以上 'This concludes (my report)' (14). The officialese indexed bureaucratic authority but did not explain the administrative thought process, thereby rendering the procedures stilted and opaque. This was noted by online viewers: 'You just directly say what you want to do' and 'What exactly is the Mainland Affairs Council saying??? [Facepalm].' Some commenters resorted to the ideology of Taiwanese ingroups versus Chinese outgroups to make sense of the policy change, with complaints such as 'Fuck. Are we Taiwanese not human?' and 'Taiwanese people are all over the place [escaping from the quarantine]. Do you still expect to rely on mainlanders?'

In light of the criticism online and from the media, the next day, the CECC commander revoked the changes and banned all Chinese spouses' children from entering Taiwan if they did not have Taiwanese nationality. In the press conference announcing the revocation, the commander stated: 我們對於這樣的一個國籍的選擇，是可以選的。那已經選擇了他的國籍，沒有選擇到台灣的國籍，那現在齁就必須要自己做安排，自己要做承擔。 'People have the option to choose their nationality. Having already chosen their nationality and not choosing Taiwanese nationality, now one will have to make their own arrangements and take the consequences.'

Discussion

The chapter investigated why the minister's account of relaxing mobility restrictions failed to generate public acceptance and support. Bruner's (1987) argument about narrative and paradigmatic reasoning offers a useful framework with which to consider the intricacies of the minister's narration and classification. The minister sought to create an ingroup identity by which the children would be aligned with Taiwan and disassociated from China. Yet there were gaps in his narration, classification, and the interplay of both communicative modes. These gaps led to not only the public reception of the children as Chinese outsiders who exploited the Taiwanese social welfare system yet did not identify with Taiwan's sovereignty but also the impression that the minister's account of the revised restriction was contradictory and bureaucratic.

In the narrative, the identity of Xiao Ming was territorialized. The minister developed Xiao Ming's character in various layers of time-space configurations. These layers were created through chronotopic contrasts between China and Taiwan. The contrasts emphasized Xiao Ming's belonging in Taiwan and his sameness to other Taiwanese children. Paradoxically, the contrasts also directed public attention to a series of social actions related to Xiao Ming's rights in Taiwan, including enrollment in Taiwanese schools and participation in the national health insurance system. These rights indexed the contentious debate in the dominant discourse regarding cross-Strait returnees' rights to social welfare, particularly when some of the returnees support China's political ideologies more vocally than they acknowledge the support they have had in Taiwan.

Furthermore, throughout the narrative, few details about the consciousness of the protagonists were given. It was not until reporters interrogated the minster during the subsequent question-and-answer time that the minster provided such details as 他的父母們都很焦慮啦 'Their parents are all very anxious' (not included in the excerpts). If good storytelling needs to simultaneously construct what characters know, think, and feel to grant the reader access into the characters' lives and minds, the narrative of Xiao Ming is insufficient.

In classification, the minister used "particularization" to exclude Chinese spouses' Chinese relatives from the restriction relaxation; he also used "categorization" to introduce the criteria for verifying the identity of the children who were permitted to return to Taiwan following the revised restriction. The discourses of particularization and categorization (Billig, 1985) embody Bruner's (1987) paradigmatic reasoning. Paradigmatic reasoning helps individuals make sense of their lived experiences by constructing a formal, objective, logico-scientific world. In this case, however, the criteria required for the children's entry into Taiwan were introduced without any details about verification procedures or supporting statistics indicating the size of the population. Instead, the criteria were enveloped in officialese that rendered the verification procedures bureaucratic and convoluted. Consequently, what seemed to be a paradigmatic discourse in fact needed concrete details for operationalizing the identity check.

Central to the analysis are the relationships between these two modes of thinking and talk. There were junctures where the modes transited or became intermingled. These junctures were overt, as in the genre-labeling 我先來講一個故事 'Let me first tell a story' (Excerpt 1) that prefaced the storytelling; they were also covert, as in the subtle switch from an address term of familiarity in Excerpt 2 (i.e., 小明 'Xiao Ming') to noun phrases of generalizability (e.g., 這些小孩 'these children') in Excerpt 3 that signaled broader referents. These junctures directed audiences' orientation to the unique frame of the information. As soon as discursive boundaries were created, gaps across the modes also became evident. When the minister introduced the entry criteria in his paradigmatic classification, his intonation and discourse marker led to the misunderstanding that the children could return to Taiwan only if they had no relative in China or if they had no relative capable of caring for them in China. The stipulation of these criteria undercut the minister's earlier narrative that Xiao Ming had gone to China with his mother to visit his grandparents. Additionally, in both modes, the minister emphasized the challenges the children encountered, including their lack of household registration, (citizen) identity, nationality, and their birth in China, but the emphasis made it difficult to understand the exact reason the children were prevented from entering Taiwan. Altogether, these gaps led to the public impression of the minister's account as inconsistent and contradictory.

Emerging research in the scholarly literature of COVID-19 discourse has uncovered the narrative construction or destruction of crisis-leadership identities, such as "strong" leaders (Jones, 2021), authentic leaders (Vásquez,

2021), and authoritative and trustworthy leaders (Seargeant, 2023). In addition to necessitating effective leadership, public health crisis communication requires government officials to create a sense of collective identity that can increase solidarity and cooperation. The findings illustrate the challenges a governmental official encountered in generating a sense of shared identity. The irrealis narrative and the paradigmatic classification were crafted to position the children as Taiwanese insiders, but the positioning was not embraced by the public; instead, the children were received as Chinese outsiders because the minister unwittingly evoked controversy over the children's nationality, which rendered restriction communication prone to politicization. To depoliticize communication, it is critical to eschew the insider-versus-outsider prejudice that easily backfires, particularly in places where geopolitical tensions are high due to enduring struggles over sovereignty. Instead, governmental officials can create a heightened sense of solidarity and cooperation by promoting inclusive identities such as common humanity-versus-intrusive virus to which the public can relate without one group becoming pitted against another.

Implication

Emergency risk communication documents such as the US Centers for Disease Control and Prevention's checklist and manual (Reynolds, 2007; Tumpey et al., 2019) operationalize effective communication in a list of do's and don'ts, e.g., "Start with empathy" and "Don't over reassure." These rules remind public health officials what to emphasize and avoid in their communication so as to create a trustworthy expert persona. This study took a different point of departure by triangulating data from the minister's official speech, journalistic questions, and public comments to understand the challenges of integrating different communicative modes into a coherent whole. The challenges included the lack of mode-specific details and the contradiction across communicative modes. These challenges debilitated official credibility and widened geopolitical fissures at a time when a sense of shared identity was urgently needed. Therefore, in addition to providing general communicative rules, emergency risk communication manuals might include mode-specific features such as metalanguage use in explaining logico-scientific evidence or reported speech in presenting narrative characters' consciousness and thus engendering public cooperation. Instead of compartmentalizing the communication into do's and don'ts, the manuals can draw attention to the relationship between different modes of communication. For example, narrative contextualizes abstract categories and paradigmatic talk classifies idiosyncrasies into generalizable categories.

Beyond narrative and paradigmatic discourses, there are other modes of communication that deserve further research attention. Especially when public health crisis communication is viewed as a two-way sense-making activity, it is not difficult to observe that all parties engage in more than one mode of communication. Government officials should not simply announce policies but also be prepared to repair gaps in communication. Journalists do not just circulate official messages but also detect inconsistencies in official messages. Public viewers are not passive consumers but active commenters on the legitimacy of official messages. The message is clear: Effective restriction communication needs to be consistent in details, complementary in modes, and congruent across individuals.

Notes

1 The official name of Taiwan is the Republic of China. "Republic of China" is used in the English translation of the transcript if this official name was used during the press conference.

2 The name "Xiao Ming" is more often used as a male name than a female name. Given this convention, I translated the pronoun "TA" in the minister's speech to the male 他 in Chinese and "he" in English although TA can be gender-neutral in spoken Chinese.

References

Anderson, B. (1983). *Imagined communities: Reflections on the origin and spread of nationalism*. Verso.

Andrée, M., Wickman, P.-O., & Lager-Nyqvist, L. (2017). Remembering as instructional work in the science classroom. In Å. Mäkitalo, P. Linell, & R. Säljö (Eds.), *Learning, interaction and the development of narrative knowing and remembering (LINT)* (pp. 75–92). Information Age Publishing.

Bakhtin, M. M. (1981). *The dialogic imagination: Four essays* (C. Emerson & M. Holquist, Trans.). University of Texas Press. (Original work published 1975)

Billig, M. (1985). Prejudice, categorization and particularization: From a perceptual to a rhetorical approach. *European Journal of Social Psychology*, *15*(1), 79–103. https://doi.org/10.1002/ejsp.2420150107

Blommaert, J., & De Fina, A. (2017). Chronotopic identities: On the timespace organization of who we are. In A. De Fina, D. Ikizoglu, & J. Wegner (Eds.), *Diversity and super-diversity: Sociocultural linguistic perspectives* (pp. 1–15). Georgetown University Press.

Briggs, C. L., & Mantini-Briggs, C. (2016). *Tell me why my children died: Rabies, indigenous knowledge, and communicative justice*. Duke University Press. https://doi.org/10.1515/9780822374398

Bruner, J. (1987). *Actual minds, possible worlds*. Harvard University Press. https://doi.org/10.2307/j.ctv26070s7

Bureau of Consular Affairs. (2020, February 10). *2月10日起經中港澳轉機得入境者，需居家檢疫14天；並限縮我國直航中港澳航線，部分機場暫停航班* [Starting from February 10, travelers transiting through China, Hong Kong, or Macau will be required to undergo 14 days of home quarantine upon entry. Additionally, direct flights between Taiwan and China, Hong Kong, and Macau will be limited, and some airports will suspend flights]. Bureau of Consular Affairs, Ministry of Foreign Affairs, Republic of China (Taiwan). www.boca.gov.tw/cp-56-5117-c83a8-1.html

Chan, H.-Y., Cheung, K. K. C., & Erduran, S. (2023). Science communication in the media and human mobility during the COVID-19 pandemic: a time series and content analysis. *Public Health*, *218*, 106–113. https://doi.org/10.1016/j.puhe.2023.03.001

De Fina, A., & Georgakopoulou, A. (2011). *Analyzing narrative: Discourse and sociolinguistic perspectives*. Cambridge University Press. https://doi.org/10.1017/CBO9781139051255

Garro, L. C., & Mattingly, C. (2001). Narrative as construct and construction. In L. C. Garro & C. Mattingly (Eds.), *Narrative and the cultural construction of illness and healing* (pp. 1–49). University of California Press.

Gibson, J., & Moran, A. (2020, April 3). *As coronavirus spreads, 'it's time to go home' Scott Morrison tells visitors and international students*. ABC News. www.abc.net.au/news/2020-04-03/coronavirus-pm-tells-international-students-time-to-go-to-home/12119568

Huang, H.-Y. (2020, March 3). 新冠肺炎防疫期間不具我國國籍陸配子女返台問題之探討 [A discussion on the issue of mainland Chinese spouses' children without Taiwanese nationality returning to Taiwan during the COVID-19 pandemic]. Legislative Yuan, Republic of China(Taiwan). www.ly.gov.tw/Pages/Detail.aspx?nodeid=6590&pid=192127

Jones, R. H. (2021). The wounded leader: The illness narratives of Boris Johnson and Donald Trump. *Discourse, context & media*, *41*, 100499. https://doi.org/10.1016/j.dcm.2021.100499

Kanno-Youngs, Z., & Semple, K. (2020, March 20). Trump Cites Coronavirus as He Announces a Border Crackdown. *The New York Times*. www.nytimes.com/2020/03/20/us/politics/trump-border-coronavirus.html

Koven, M. (2019). Narrating desire for place: Chronotopes of desire for the Portuguese homeland before and after "Return." In R. Piazza (Ed.), *Discourses of identity in liminal places and spaces* (pp. 42–63). Routledge. https://doi.org/10.4324/9781351183383-3

Lee, S. -H. (2020). The dialectical unfolding of paradigmatic and narrative thinking in a Chinese-as-a-foreign-language classroom. *Classroom Discourse*, *11*(4), 316–336. https://doi.org/10.1080/19463014.2019.1633550

Li, C. N., & Thompson, S. A. (1981). *Mandarin Chinese: A functional reference grammar*. University of California Press.

Lin, H.-C., & Chung, J. (2016, March 11). Huang An returns for medical care. *Taipei Times*. www.taipeitimes.com/News/front/archives/2016/03/11/2003641297

Ochs, E., Taylor, C., Rudolph, D., & Smith, R. (1992). Storytelling as a theory-building activity. *Discourse Processes*, *15*(1), 37–72. https://doi.org/10.1080/01638539209544801

Peterson, S. M. (2009). Narrative and paradigmatic explanations in preschool science discourse. *Discourse Processes*, *46*(4), 369–399. https://doi.org/10.1080/01638530902959448

Pomerantz, A. (1986). Extreme case formulations: A way of legitimizing claims. *Human Studies*, *9*(2/3), 219–229. www.jstor.org/stable/20008968

Reynolds, B. (2007). *Crisis and emergency risk communication: Pandemic influenza*. https://stacks.cdc.gov/view/cdc/7037

Seargeant, P. (2023). *Crisis leadership: Boris Johnson and political persuasion during the COVID pandemic*. Cambridge University Press. https://doi.org/10.1017/9781009321983

Taiwan Centers for Disease Control (2020, September 23). *Starting from September 24, Mainland Chinese spouses may apply to enter Taiwan*. Taiwan Centers for

Disease Control. www.cdc.gov.tw/En/Bulletin/Detail/3LlCYr67CVXx--6UQMLWJQ?typeid=158

Tsai, C.-H. (2023). 臺灣對兩岸社會交流規範之國族認同建構：以新冠疫情下民進黨政府對兩岸人員往來的管制為例 [The construction of national identity in Taiwan's regulation on cross-strait social interflows: Taking DPP government's control of cross-strait personnel exchanges under the COVID-19 pandemic as example]. *Chinese Political Science Review*, *75*, 1–40. https://doi.org/10.6229/CPSR.202306_(75).0001

Tsao, F.-N., & Guo, W. (2020, October 5). 愛在瘟疫蔓延時——封關8個月，扛著時代巨石的兩岸家庭 [Love in times of epidemic, eight months of border closures: Cross-Strait families carrying heavy burden of time]. The Reporter. www.twreporter.org/a/cross-strait-marriage-during-covid-19-lockdown

Tumpey, A. J., Daigle, D., & Nowak, G. (2019). Communicating during an outbreak or public health investigation. In S. A. Rasmussen & R. A. Goodman (Eds.), *The CDC field epidemiology manual* (pp. 243–260). Oxford University Press. https://doi.org/10.1093/oso/9780190933692.001.0001

Vásquez, C. (2021). Leading with stories: Andrew Cuomo, family narratives and authentic leadership. *Discourse, Context & Media*, *41*, 100507. https://doi.org/10.1016/j.dcm.2021.100507

Wald, P. (2008). *Contagious: Cultures, carriers, and the outbreak narrative*. Duke University Press. https://doi.org/10.1515/9780822390572

Yang, H.-J. (2021). 疫情是種族歧視的一面照妖鏡：新住民與新二代面臨的困境與臺灣社會應有的省思 [The pandemic is a way of revealing racial discrimination: The challenges faced by new immigrants and the new second generation and the call for introspection in Taiwanese society]. *Humanities & Social Sciences Briefing*, *22*(3), 6–11. www.nstc.gov.tw/nstc/attachments/563ceda4-364a-4b17-9b54-30956a772be1

Yeung, J. (2022, May 13). *China tightens ban on 'non-essential' overseas travel as lockdown anger rises*. CNN. https://edition.cnn.com/2022/05/13/china/china-covid-outbound-travel-restriction-intl-hnk-mic/index.html

4 Numerical Classification

The day was bound to come. In May 2021, Taiwan faced its first large community outbreak of COVID-19. The outbreak jolted the public and health officials because, throughout 2020, Taiwan had maintained a state of relative normalcy, with a daily case number in the single digits, if not zero, even as many places worldwide were being ravaged by the pandemic.

Now, the outbreak was swelling throughout the island. The speed of reporting could not keep up with the rapidly increasing daily case number. As a result, the official statistics no longer reflected the latest pandemic conditions. In an effort to restore their appearance of control over the situation, public health officials needed to clear a backlog of unreported cases and provide the public with the revised case numbers at press conferences. How, if at all, did they explain the revisions to the public, and were they successful? Would the officials encounter pushback from the journalists and the public over their revisions?

In this chapter, I draw on an episode of introducing data revisions to illustrate that numbers are not only for quantifying the speed and degree of an outbreak but also for qualitatively annotating the outbreak. Throughout the chapter, I use statistics, numbers, and data interchangeably to refer to quantitative representations. Numbers take on qualitative meanings through classification that sorts numerical tokens into categorical types. I illustrate this token-type relationship in my analysis of the Taiwanese Central Epidemic Command Center (CECC) commander's speech, in which the commander classified the revised numbers into the categorical type of *retrospective adjustment*, defined as the practice of attributing unreported backlogged cases to the dates that these cases should have been reported. The category provoked public support and criticism. To quell the public criticism, the commander contextualized the revised numbers using narratives, graphs, gestures, and metadiscourse. The contextualization aggregated and disaggregated the numbers to form different numerical patterns and categorical relations, which in turn enabled the commander to communicate official control over the outbreak's progression and the fleetingness of time. These qualities of numerical classification suggest that numbers are not just decontextualized variables

DOI: 10.4324/9781003545002-4

or representative of cold logicality. Instead, through classification, numbers are infused with meanings and set in relation to past, present, and hypothetical time. However, it is through these qualitative meanings that numbers become open to reinterpretation and even contestation.

This chapter takes an interdisciplinary approach. My analysis of numerical classification is motivated by anthropological, communicative, and sociological research on numbers in contextualized practices (e.g., Bowker & Starr, 1999; Lawson, 2023; Stafford, 2009); numerical rhetoric in discourse analysis (e.g., Billig, 2021; van Dijk, 2018); social interactional approaches to speech genres (e.g., De Fina & Georgakopoulou, 2011; Gordon, 2023; Ochs & Capps, 2001); and the interface of language and cognition through embodied experience (e.g., Goodwin, 2018; Lakoff & Johnson, 1980). Each enterprise is grounded in its own unique epistemologies about communication in society that inform its analytic foci. However, the approaches share an emphasis on the creation or representation of meaning through language or multimodalities. In this chapter, I synthesize the analytical strengths of these meaning-based theories and research to uncover linguistic and multimodal features of numerical classification. To achieve this goal, I triangulate various data sources: transcribed sequences of the public health officials' press conference, graphs created and used by the commander to account for the data revisions, and comments left by public online viewers. The triangulation reveals a constellation of semiotic resources that the commander used to shape the social perception of the pandemic outbreak.

In what follows, I first define the concept of numerical classification by drawing on examples and theories in different disciplines. I then provide contextual information about how the number of daily COVID-19 cases was produced and reported in Taiwan before and during the large community outbreak. Subsequently, I show that the commander used what I call *numbers talk* to highlight that numbers convey more than what they appear to show. I then analyze how the commander showed the qualitative meanings of numbers through numerical classification in narrative, graphs, gestures, and metadiscourse. I also attend to the metaphors through which the commander responded to public criticism of the classification. I conclude the chapter by summarizing the findings and offering practical implications.

Numerical Classification

My analysis is based on the notion of numerical classification, defined as the process of aggregating or disaggregating numbers according to categorical types. Numbers are cultural tools that humans rely upon to gain control over diverse experiences by converting idiosyncrasies into comparable symbols. Seen more critically, numbers abstract and dehumanize experiences. The news coverage of pandemic outbreaks demonstrates how numbers can make events that seem temporally and spatially distant more comparable and relatable. When reporting on the dire situation of the COVID-19 pandemic, many media outlets turned to history to compare the numbers of lives lost from the outbreak with those lost during other traumatic events. For instance, the headline "New York State's Coronavirus Deaths Now More Than Double 9/11 Fatalities" appeared in the *Los Angeles Times* (Finnegan, 2020), and *200,000 People Have Died From Covid-19 in the US. That's More Than the US Battle Deaths From 5 Wars Combined* was featured on *CNN* (Yan, 2020).

These news headlines suggest that numbers play an important role in shaping individuals' perceptions and imagination of a crisis. When numbers are used as meaningful ways to engage in and think about a certain phenomenon, they bound the phenomenon by representing it. Lawson (2023) calls this process a ***data bound***. For example, case numbers play a key role in determining whether infectious diseases are viewed as global, national, or regional phenomena and stratifying the position of nation-states according to the health of their populations (Briggs & Mantini-Briggs, 2003).

Numbers are not static symbols. Numbers become malleable through arithmetic operations such as addition and subtraction or multiplication and division. To classify numbers is to apply arithmetic operations according to categorical types. Consider the example of COVID-19 case numbers. The numbers of COVID-19 cases from diverse places can be combined to account for the category of daily COVID-19 cases in a nation. The numbers of daily confirmed cases can be disaggregated to instantiate specific categories such as age and gender. As such, numbers are a powerful means of naturalizing categories in a society (Bowker & Starr, 1999). Numerical classification is a process of mapping numerical tokens with categorical types to represent or, put more accurately, construct realities.

Numerical classification creates relations and patterns. Bruner (1987, p. 12) argued that in classification, "categories are established, instantiated, idealized, and related one to the other to form a system." Such relations are created not only among categories but also among the numbers that instantiate categorical types. For instance, numbers have numerous inherent relations, including predecessors and successors, ordinal and cardinal numbers, as well as precise and round numbers. Numbers also constitute patterns when they are structured according to a temporal order (such as in a pandemic outbreak curve) or used in scoring that evaluates objects or individuals on a scale of "better or worse" or "more or less" (Mau, 2019) that yields a pattern of hierarchies (such as in global university rankings). When patterns and relations become recognizable, they attract qualitative judgments and accumulate value. For example, one might say that "successfully" flattening an epidemiological curve indicates "good" governance. As such, numbers are infused with evaluative qualities through the patterns and relations created during classification.

To say that numbers have qualitative meanings is not to deny that numbers can function as a starting point for objectivity and precision in modern science. Instead, it is to highlight that, like other communicative means, numbers can be aggregated or disaggregated to achieve speakers' communicative goals: in other words, quantities can be manipulated to communicate qualities. Billig's

(2021) critical discourse analysis showed that during the COVID-19 pandemic, senior members of the British government used round numbers to set goals and underscore official achievements, but these round numbers became incentives for manipulating the production of more precise numbers. van Dijk (2018) used the term "numbers game" to describe the rhetorical moves of emphasis and hyperbole. He showed that the immigration discourse of right-wing politicians and journalists is replete with numbers, and these numbers serve the rhetorical function of emphasizing the dangers of immigration. Right-wing media particularly tend to present the numbers and their consequences as facts without alethic modalities, e.g., "suggest," "probably," and "may." Clearly, numbers can be socially and politically charged.

Numbers also exist qualitatively in everyday life. Stafford's ethnographic study (2009) indicated that numbers figure prominently in life-accounting and self-imaging in Taiwan. Stafford showed that for ordinary people in real-world contexts, numbers are not neutral tools strictly for calculation and counting. Instead, numbers are central to folk understanding of realities because numbers have value, as in profit and loss calculation. Numbers are also about the fatefulness of human experience. Numbers are often used to interpret the logic of the universe and help individuals imagine themselves as part of it. Because of their qualitative association with value, fate, and logic, numbers can help people understand, control, and even change the course of their lives and the world around them (Stafford, 2020).

In this chapter, I contribute to discussions about the social perception of a public health crisis (Briggs & Mantini-Briggs, 2003; Lawson, 2023); numerical rhetoric (Billig, 2021; van Dijk, 2018); and qualitative mathematics in Taiwan (Stafford, 2009, 2020). My purpose in studying numerical classification is not to repeat the argument that numbers have qualitative meanings. Instead, I seek to understand *how* numbers derive their qualitative meanings through patterns and relations created during classification.

Context

Before the Outbreak

Before delving into the context of the episode analyzed in this chapter, it is important to know how daily case numbers were calculated and presented in Taiwan prior to the large community outbreak in May 2021. Before the outbreak, all COVID-19 cases were confirmed through COVID-19 polymerase chain reaction (PCR) tests. Pathologists' caseload was manageable because Taiwan was able to keep most of its COVID-19 cases offshore, and Taiwan did not conduct mass testing on all of its citizens. The results of the PCR tests were required to be uploaded to the Laboratory Information Management System (LIMS) and Infectious Disease Announce System (IDAS) hosted by the Taiwan Centers for Disease Control within 24 hours of test completion (Yen & Kung, 2021). To calculate the total number of daily cases, public health officials used the date that each positive PCR result was interpreted by pathologists (Chen, 2021). That is, daily case numbers were calculated based on PCR confirmation dates, not testing dates or symptom onset dates.

A daily case number was presented to the public at a COVID-19 press conference livestreamed online at 2:00 p.m. every day. At the start of each conference, the commander announced the number in performative utterances (Austin, 1962) that brought into being a new pandemic situation: for instance, the commander might say 今天要宣佈我們新增了9例確診 'Today I announce that we have an increase of 9 new confirmed cases.' Watching the daily press conference and waiting for the commander's announcement of the total number of cases became a daily routine for many Taiwanese people (Chen, 2020). The tone of the conferences fluctuated according to the number of daily cases. An announcement of zero cases was celebrated and desired by all. The officials showed their elation about zero cases through a creative display of local fish and produce at such conferences. The fish was associated with zero through homophones: for example, there was a display of groupers with the sign of 以石慶十、十全十美 'Use groupers [*shi*ban] to celebrate 10 [*shi*] successive days of zero case, perfect in every way.' The produce was associated with zero because of its shape: the shape of a guava or a watermelon resembles a zero. Figure 4.1 shows the eight guavas that were sitting on the table as the commander announced the eighth day of zero instances of local infection. This rendition of daily case numbers distinguished Taiwan, in quantity and

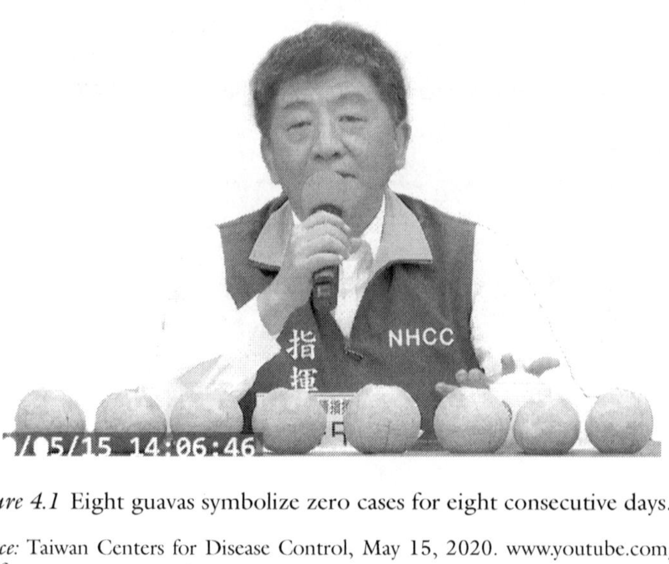

Figure 4.1 Eight guavas symbolize zero cases for eight consecutive days.

Source: Taiwan Centers for Disease Control, May 15, 2020. www.youtube.com/watch?v=6p65hh2lftg

quality, from the rest of the world that was trapped in a cycle of lockdowns and reopenings. The announcement of the daily case number also inculcated a sense of the ineffable power of numbers in prompting affective reactions and creating different realities.

During the Outbreak

Taiwan officially entered the phase of a large community outbreak and remained in this status from May 19 to July 26, 2021. During this time, the CECC categorized the outbreak as a Level 3 crisis emergency, which is defined as either more than three clusters of community infections in a week or more than ten confirmed local cases with unknown infectious sources in one day. Under the emergency classification, individuals were permitted to go outside but were required to wear masks. Additionally, there was a limit on the number of individuals attending an outdoor or indoor gathering. Only essential businesses were allowed to operate.

During the outbreak, all positive cases of COVID-19 needed to be confirmed through lab reports, such as PCR tests and clinical evidence. The daily case number was announced at 2:00 p.m. every day. COVID-19 rapid antigen tests were used in some places to screen for individuals who should receive PCR testing (Yen & Kung, 2021). Furthermore, daily case numbers were presented in graphical form, not just verbally. No produce or fish was on display; this was only for the days in 2020 when there were no known cases of local infection.

The data that I use to illustrate numerical classification consists of a 71-minute video of the press conference on May 22, 2021, and 15,763 live-chat comments about the conference made by public online viewers. The conference was held during the large community outbreak. I focus on the conference held on May 22 because during the conference, the commander introduced the neologism 校正回歸 'retrospective adjustment' to account for a portion of the COVID-19 cases reported that day. The reporting of these cases was delayed because at the height of the outbreak, there was a large backlog of PCR tests waiting for pathological interpretation and lags in uploading the PCR results to the LIMS and the IDAS of the Taiwan Centers for Disease Control. As the speed was gradually ramped up and the backlog was cleared, officials attributed previously unreported cases to the dates that these cases should have been reported (i.e., the PCR confirmation dates). The commander called this practice of data revision retrospective adjustment. That is, retrospective adjustment is simultaneously a process and a category.

The introduction of the category provoked both controversy and support. Some online commenters expressed confusion when seeing or hearing the announcement of the category along with the associated number, asking 'What the heck is retrospective adjustment?' and 'Is this a numbers game?

What is meant by 400 cases of retrospective adjustment?' Others sarcastically commented on the neologism: '(We) have a new term again' and 'Shih-chung Chen [the name of the commander], the term inventor.' However, other online commenters echoed the officials' justification of the category, writing 'At least (the officials are) not hiding cases.' Still others challenged other viewers' criticism of the neologism, writing 'Go back to school, OK? The term already exists' and 'Those (people) who are still asking about retrospective adjustment. Are they illiterate?'

The introduction of retrospective adjustment fractured the online audience into supporters and opponents. The controversy of retrospective adjustment is also shown in its high social volume online, i.e., the total number of mentions across social media. According to Daileyview (2022), an online media outlet that surveys online forums using big-data analytics, retrospective adjustment ranked first among the commander's utterances during the pandemic because it had the highest social volume online. High volume is not necessarily good or bad; it merely indicates the amount of attention that something has received online. However, high attention is oftentimes associated with topics or issues that evoke polarized responses from the public. To fully understand the reasons for the polarization, it is imperative to investigate the discourse surrounding this numerical classification.

Analysis

In this section, I present my multimodal discourse analysis of the commander's introduction of retrospective adjustment as a new classificatory category. I start with an analysis of numbers talk, which underscores the message that the commander sought to convey about numbers. I then take an in-depth look at the commander's use of narratives, graphs, gestures, and metadiscourse to infuse numbers with different qualitative meanings. Finally, I analyze the metaphors used by others to criticize the classification and the commander's response to these criticisms, which involved reframing the metaphors.

Numbers Talk

Numeracy is central to the interpretation of pandemic conditions. Numbers are more than the objects they purport to measure. They create "powerful imaginings of society and our place within it" (Briggs & Mantini-Briggs, 2003, pp. 266–267). During the press conference, the commander was aware of the rich meaning that numbers could have in communicating the outbreak status. He repeatedly used numbers talk to transform numbers into discursive objects for comments, explanations, and clarifications. Numbers talk suggests that numbers have meanings other than the mathematic or arithmetic reasoning they represent. Below are the commander's numbers talk produced throughout the conference:

- 這個數字不是大家就這樣看看就欸今天高高低低，不是這個．這數字有它代表的一個曲線的意義

  'The number is not just for everyone to view casually. Like today is high or low. It is not like this. The number's meaning is represented through a curve.'

- 我再強調這數字是要代表實情嘛. ...真正的情況

  'I would like to emphasize again. The number should represent realities. … Real situations.'

- 每一個數目字都代表每一個病人

  'Each figure represents each patient.'

- 齁所以不是一個數目字啦齁 這不是新台幣這是人啦齁

  'Hm so it's not a figure hm. This is not the New Taiwanese Dollar. This is a human being hm.'

- 這數字不是只有看這個數字. ... 齁它要傳達一個數字所代表的意義. ..那這個數字才有意義

  'The number is not just for viewing. Hm it needs to convey the meaning that the number represents. Only then is the number meaningful.'

To help the public see that there was more to the numbers than it seemed, the commander contextualized the numbers and their classifications using at least four different semiotic means: narrative, graphs, gestures, and metadiscourse. Each semiotic means highlights an aspect of the revised numbers, including problem-solving, reversible time, the irrealis, and the realis. In what follows, I contextualize each semiotic means by first introducing its relevant theories or constructs and then analyzing the corresponding press conference sequences.

Narrative of Successful Problem-Solving

In the eyes of the commander, revised numbers represented official successes in problem-solving. This view was shown through the commander's use of narrative. In this context, narrative is a speech genre and social practice that endows lived experience with order and meaning (De Fina & Georgakopoulou, 2011; Ochs & Capps, 2001). A problem-solving narrative was used by the commander to structure the officials' experience of handling the backlog. This type of narrative helps make an experience highly tellable because it involves problems that affect everyone and need to be solved.

Excerpt 1 illustrates the embedding of numerical classifications within the narrative of problem-solving. In the narrative, the commander characterized the numbers as the outcome of having successfully solved the backlog problem.

Excerpt 1

1	Commander	...那前兩天呢大家也= ..注意到, ..就是說其實我們這個整個的, ...齁採檢在最主要是在報告這一端, ..齁其實就=, ..產生了塞車的情況.	Hm about two days ago, everyone also noticed, I mean, that actually our whole hm testing, primarily in the (case) reporting end, hm actually already, has a backlog of cases.
2		...(.9)所以從那天開始我們也齁, 積極地齁, 來研究怎麼樣<MRC簡化MRC>, ..齁相關的一個通報的<HI程序HI>,那希望它能夠齁, 速度能夠加快.	So starting from that date, we also hm proactively hm researched how to simplify hm relevant procedures for reporting. Hoping it can- hm the (reporting) speed can become faster.
3		齁讓我們對於整個的疫情的研判, ..齁能夠更及時. ..齁那經過這幾天的一個改善. 齁那就...把這個通報的速度齁, 把它大為提升. ..齁大為提升.	Hm so that we can assess the whole pandemic situation. Hm (the assessment) can be more timely. Hm hm after the improvement in the (past) couple days, hm then, (we) greatly enhanced the reporting speed. Greatly enhanced.
4		...那在昨天因為在效率的提升, 所以昨天我們大概也清了大概1萬多件的齁, ..的一些舊案. ...(.7)齁那然後呢這裡面齁, ..有400個, ..齁有400個案例. ..齁有400個案例.	Hm yesterday because of the enhanced efficiency, yesterday we cleaned up about more than ten thousand cases hm. (They are) some old cases. Hm then inside (these cases) hm, there are 400. Hm there are 400 cases. Hm there are 400 cases.

As shown in Excerpt 1, the storytelling began with the commander's account of the backlog in reporting confirmed cases (1). The commander presented the problem by using the indefinite pronoun of 大家 'everyone' coupled with the sense verb of 注意 'notice' to downgrade the unexpectedness of the problem, thereby making the problem controllable and solvable. The commander subsequently used the collective pronoun 我們 'we' to introduce the officials as the protagonists. Their determination to resolve the problem was positively cast using the manner adverb 積極地 'proactively' and openly disclosed through the mental verb 希望 'hoping' (2). Finally, problems were successfully solved as indicated by the booster (大為 'greatly' line 3), the actions (提升 'enhanced' line 3 and 清了 'clean up' line 4), and the numbers (1萬多件 'more than ten thousand' and '400' line 4). More specifically, the commander instantiated official efforts in the round number (1萬多件 'about more than ten thousand' line 4) and achievements in the precise number ('400' line 4). Note that the commander did not share the total sum of backlogged cases. In this way, he avoided giving the impression that the officials had not yet fully resolved the backlog and thus were still not in full control of the situation. The selective use of numbers enabled the commander to grasp and communicate the seemingly uncontrollable outbreak. Presenting revised numbers in the problem-solving narrative imparted positive qualities to the quantities.

Graph of Reversible Time

When case numbers are interpreted according to pandemic time, these numbers become powerful symbols that can shape the perception and imagination of the outbreak's progression. One classificatory principle of retrospective adjustment is reversible time. That is, previously announced case numbers can be retrospectively adjusted. When returning to previous time to adjust the numbers, time is conceptualized as intervals, not a cut-off point. A histogram is a "phenomenal object" (Goodwin, 2018) that animates the work and discourse of epidemiology in conceptualizing the relationship between time intervals and case numbers. In Figure 4.2, the commander used a graph to present case numbers in reversible time intervals.

Figure 4.3 shows the graph, which contains a table and a histogram. The Taiwan Centers for Disease Control (Taiwan CDC) authorized the use of the graph in this chapter on the condition that their English-language annotation and translation were adopted instead of mine. I have included their annotation and translation in red. I also parenthesized some of their English translation to show the English meaning that was not clearly or explicitly conveyed through the Chinese characters in the graph. The endnotes of the chapter include Taiwan CDC's further explanation[1] about the graph and definition[2] of 研判日 in the graph that has the literal meaning of 'interpretation date' but was translated as 'the date of being identified as COVID-19' according to Taiwan CDC's request. The English annotation and translation indicate Taiwan CDC's emphasis on the 'processed backlog.'

As Figure 4.3 shows, the table had numbers tabulated in columns with headings that identified the unit of classification (i.e., date) and categorical types (i.e., initially published case number and case number including the processed backlog). The histogram plotted the number of COVID-19 cases per day. Along the *x*-axis were time intervals starting from May 1 and extending to May 22. Along the *y*-axis were the numbers of confirmed cases. Through the color and height of the upright bars, the histogram visualized the numbers of published cases, processed backlog cases, and aggregated cases every day.

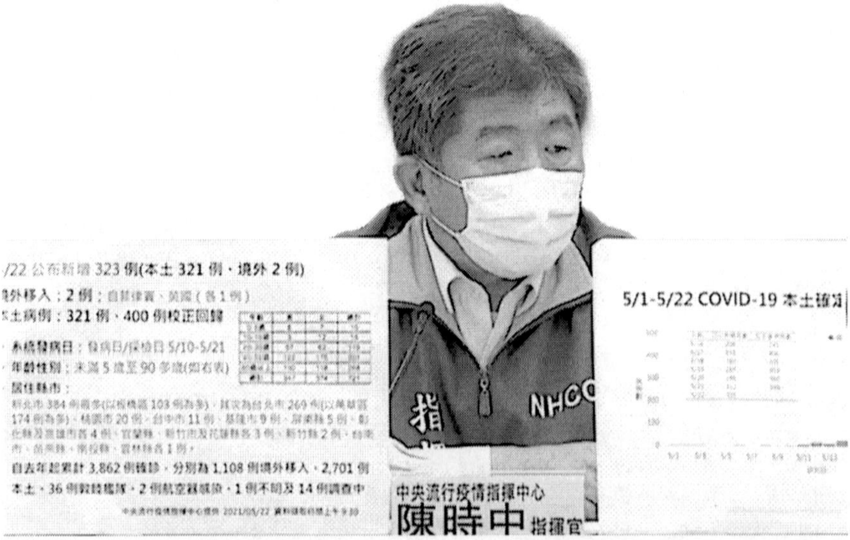

Figure 4.2 The commander presented a graph to illustrate retrospective adjustment.

Source: Taiwan Centers for Disease Control, May 22, 2021. www.youtube.com/watch?v=5oqunnTeh3Q

Together, the data visualizations illustrate how numbers were aggregated and disaggregated to create patterns (i.e., an outbreak curve) that enabled public health officials to see the peak and trough of the outbreak. More importantly, the visualizations naturalized the category of retrospective adjustment by juxtaposing it with other categories.

Data visualizations are material artifacts created for conveying official messages. To analyze tools without understanding how they are used in practice would be to overlook the real-time use of numerical classification. Excerpt 2 shows how the commander introduced Figure 4.3 through talk.

Excerpt 2

1	Commander	...(.9)那另外在大家的右手邊是我們昨天整體齁, ..在速度加快通報, ..然後把它清查出來, ..在前一段時間, ...齁等於是一個塞車的案子.	and also, on everyone's right-hand side are (cases that) yesterday, we enhanced the overall speed of reporting and identified (these COVID-19 cases). For a period of time in the past- (These) are backlog cases.

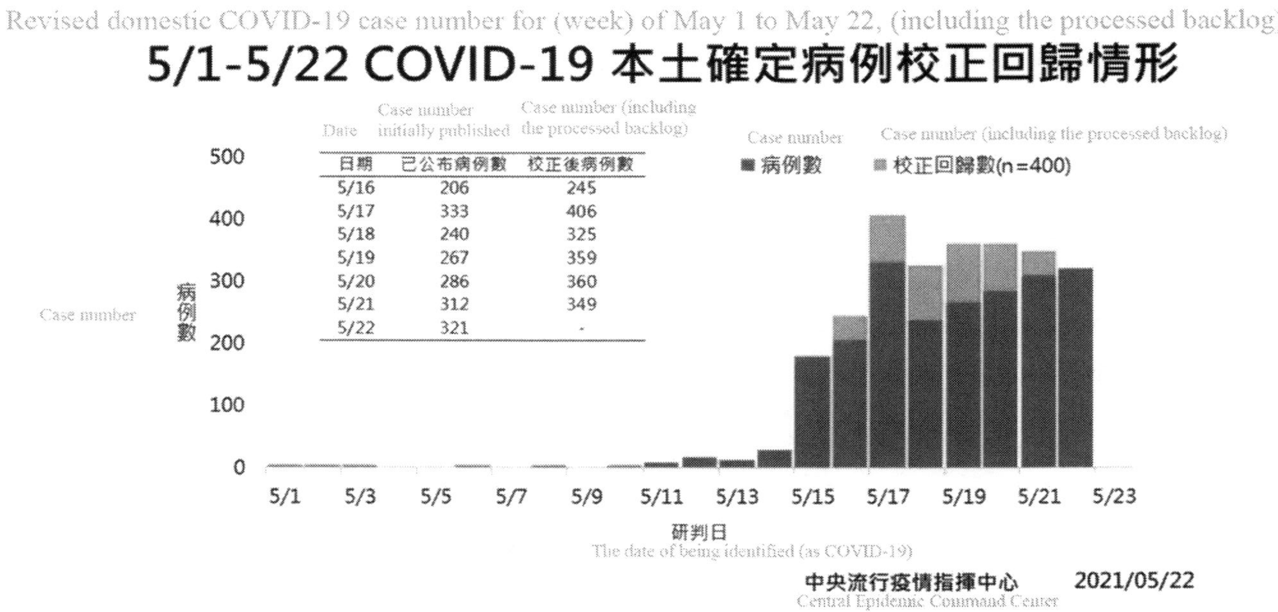

Figure 4.3 Visualizations of retrospective adjustment.

Source: Graph by the Taiwan Central Epidemic Command Center and used with permission from the Taiwan Centers for Disease Control. www.youtube.com/watch?v=5oqunnTeh3Q

2	...那因為它是一個塞車的案子要讓這樣的一個疫情能夠看得更清楚, ...齁所以我們就把它校正回歸到, 齁原來它應該要被通報出來如果沒有塞車的情況下.	Hm because they are backlog cases. To make this kind of pandemic situation clearer to see, hm so we retrospectively adjusted the cases hm back to how they should have been reported if there had been no backlog.
3	...(.9)齁所以會從5月<A16 17 18 19 A> 20 ... 21, 齁都做了校正. ...(.7)那整體看這樣的一個齁, 圖表來看, ...齁那事實上還是在, ..欸5月17號,	Hm so (we) would make hm adjustments from May 16, to 17, to 18, to 19, to 20, and to 21. Hm viewing as a whole in this kind of a hm graph. Hm hm in fact, it is still hm on May 17 that
4	...齁這時候的病例數<MRC會最多MRC>. ...齁會最多.	Hm this date has the most cases. Hm (this date) has the most cases.

In Excerpt 2, the commander directed the audience's attention to reversible time as captured in the graph. He started by characterizing the newly tallied confirmed cases as a backlog (1) and then justified the classification through the deontic modality of 應該 'should' (2). The commander subsequently emphasized reversible time by temporally conditioning the classification in the direction 從 'from'; the intervals 5月16 17 18 19 20 ... 21 'May 16, to 17, to 18, to 19, to 20, and to 21'; and reversibility 做了校正 'make hm adjustment' (3). Because each date was linked to a numerical value, the dates became comparable, not just chronological. That is, May 17 was topicalized in a construction that coupled the superlative 最多 'the most' with a repetition and the prosody of careful enunciation (4). By integrating these linguistic, discursive, and prosodic features, the commander made salient the relationship between case numbers and time intervals in the histogram, which is the defining feature of retrospective adjustment.

Gesture of the Irrealis

Following the presentation of retrospective adjustment, the commander took journalists' questions about the numerical classification. He strove to defend the classification with the resources at hand, including by disproving a journalist's proposed classification through his gestures toward the irrealis. Irrealis descriptions introduce a particular display of numbers under a hypothetical condition. In Mandarin Chinese, the irrealis can be created through the hypothetical conjunction 如果 'if,' e.g., 我們就把它校正回歸到, 齁原來它應該要被通報出來如果沒有塞車的情況下 'We retrospectively adjusted the cases hm back to how they should have been reported if there had been no backlog.' As Excerpt 3 shows, the irrealis was multimodally constructed by the commander, whose gestures visualized the alternative aggregation of numbers proposed by the journalist to counter the official classification.

Excerpt 3

1	Journalist	..今天我們增加回歸的這400例, ...就大家還是蠻疑惑的, 為什麼我們就不直接講說就是新增700是擔心大家會- ...<A因為聽到這個數字A>而嚇到嗎.	Today we have 400 cases of retrospective adjustment. Everyone is still quite confused. Why can't we just directly say it is a new addition of 700 cases? Is it because of the worry that everyone will be scared when hearing the number?
2		((omitting turns about other questions))	
3	Commander	好這個病例為什麼要回歸啦齁. ...這個數字不是大家就這樣看看就欸今天高高低低, 不是這個. 這數字有它代表的一個曲線的意義.	OK why did (we) retrospectively adjust the numbers? The number is not just for everyone to view casually. Like today is high or low. It is not like this. The number's meaning is represented through a curve.
4		...齁如果你把這樣的一個行政上面的案例, ..把它歸在這上面, ...那你會造成很大的一個誤解.	Hm if you (sort) these kinds of administrative cases- sort them into this, you would then bring about a very big misinterpretation.

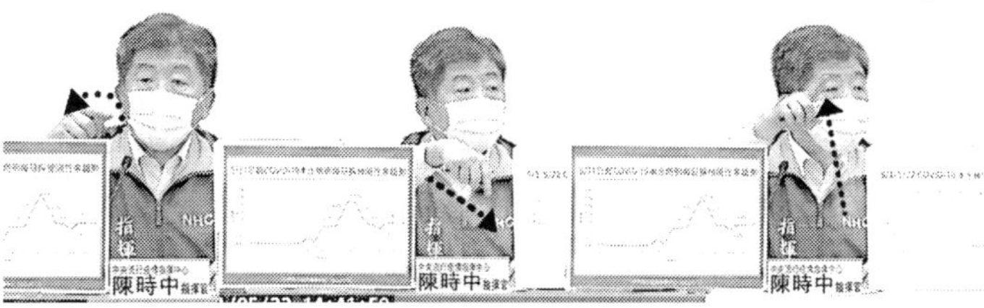

5		那對於疫情的一個判斷, ...是非常不利的.	That is ... very disadvantageous to the assessment of the pandemic situation.

In Excerpt 3, the commander responded to the journalist's question and speculation about the psychological impact of a cumulative total on the public (1). His response emphasized the importance of understanding the curve of COVID-19 positive rates and its implications for public health measures (3). To prove the journalist's proposed aggregation to be false, he engaged everyone in the irrealis through the hypothetical conjunction of 如果 'if' and the indefinite second-person pronoun of 你 'you' (4). Imagistically, his index finger improvised a graph in the air (4), which specified and instantiated the hypothetical scenarios constructed through his talk. That is, he first drew a circle to metaphorically represent the backlogged cases described in his speech as 這樣的 'these kinds.' His hand then moved forward toward the graph that he used to represent retrospective adjustment, and his index finger pointed down to a spot in front of him. The forward movement and downward motion made concrete the aggregation of all COVID-19 cases to a particular date in the graph, which was also specified by the demonstrative pronoun 這 'this' in his speech. Subsequently, his hand dramatically moved upward, as did his index finger. The upward movement iconically represented the height of the bars in the bar graph and instantiated the misinterpretation that was left unspecified in his speech as 很大的一個誤解 'a very big misinterpretation.' In the end, the commander negatively valorized the journalist's numerical aggregation: 非常不利的 'very disadvantageous' (5). Thus, gestures visualized numerical patterns under hypothetical time, and the patterns were valorized as misleading.

Metadiscourse of the Realis

Metadiscourse is a discourse about discourse (Gordon, 2023). It serves multiple purposes in communicating crisis classifications, including enacting biomedical authority and animating adversarial comments (Lee, 2024). The journalists at the press conference relied on metadiscourse to present their pointed questions and push for newsworthy categories. For example, during the conference, some of the journalists asked 為什麼我們就不直接講說就是新增700? 'Why can't we just directly say an increase of 700 new cases?' and 那因為有媒體直接寫說今日單日新增了 700例, 那想問一下我們是不是可以統一這樣寫? 'Uh because some media directly wrote today there is an increase of 700 new cases in a day, uh I would like to ask if we can uniformly write like this.' The officials also used metadiscourse to defend their classification of case numbers as representing the realis. Excerpt 4 illustrates this push-and-pull (see also Chapter 2) involved in presenting the pandemic numbers in metadiscourse.

Excerpt 4

1	Journalist	那想問這個400例的回歸是不是全- ..世界, ..台灣首創的名詞謝謝.	Hm (I) would like to ask if the 400 cases of retrospective (adjustment)- Is Taiwan the first in the whole- world to initiate the use of this term? Thanks.

2		((omitting official replies to other questions))	
3	Commander	在做這樣的一個不管是流行病學或在公共衛生或者政策也好. ...我再強調這數字是要代表實情嘛. ...真正的情況.	To make this kind of- Whether it is in epidemiology, public health, or policy, I (would like to) emphasize again. The number should represent realities. Real situations.
4		...齁比如我們來講說那5月- ...齁比如說5月17號我們是333例嗎? 不是.	Hm for example, let's say May- hm for example, say May 17. Do we have 333 cases? No.
5		..5月33號- 5月17號我們是406例. ...(.7)齁這是發生的, ..齁在那一天所發生的數目. 那重要是這個正確性.	On May 33- May 17, we have 406 cases. Hm this is (what) happened. Hm the (case) number of the day. Hm what is important is the accuracy.
6		...齁不在於就是說原來因為塞車所影響的這樣的一個數目. ...(.7)齁那樣對我們整體對疫情的掌控跟判斷是沒有意義的.	Hm not the (overall backlog case) number due to the initial delay. Hm that is meaningless to our overall control and interpretation about the pandemic situation.
7		...所以任何在上面調查也好, ...那有這些數目上的一個排序的錯誤, 那是一定要把它校正的.	So any investigation based on it. If there are errors about arranging the numbers in order, it must be corrected.

In Excerpt 4, the journalist criticized the validity of the numerical classification through the extreme case formulation (Pomerantz, 1986) 全世界 'the whole world.' (1). The metadiscursive referent 名詞 'term' (1) indicated that the trouble source is the referential form of the category 回歸 'retrospective adjustment.' The commander responded with the metadiscursive operator 強調 'emphasize' to buttress his previous proposition that numbers should represent realities (3); he also used the juxtaposition of the metadiscursive operator 比如說 'for example' and verb 講說 'say' to instantiate what such realities should and should not be like (4). Different types of numerical reasoning were then qualitatively evaluated. That is, numerical disaggregation based on successive time was 重要 'important' (5), whereas the cumulative total of all backlogged COVID-19 cases (i.e., the journalist's characterization) was 沒有意義的 'meaningless' (6). In other words, the commander indicated that numbers are only meaningful and reflect realities when they are disaggregated according to a temporal order.

Contested Classifications in Metaphor

The classification was not without controversy. It recreated relations and patterns based on (dis)aggregated numbers. For the public and journalists, if numbers could be adjusted after their publication, patterns and relations could also be recreated, and all previous performative announcements about daily case numbers became void. Revising publicized numbers thus triggered a chain of changes.

The commander's introduction of the classification quickly provoked online speculation about underreporting. These instances of speculation were framed with conventional metaphors related to accounting and poker games. These metaphors created a coherent network of entailments that highlighted certain aspects of experiences and obscured others (Lakoff & Johnson, 1980). In other words, the use of metaphors simultaneously afforded and constrained individuals to think about the classification in specific ways.

Following the introduction of retrospective adjustment to classify case numbers, online viewers adopted the poker-game metaphor of 蓋牌 'folding cards' to express their belief that the officials had covered up the truth about the pandemic. They used phrases such as 'fold it well. fold it fully,' 'secretively folding cards,' and 'folding 400 cases. Is it very difficult to understand?' Supporters of the classification dismissed the speculation: 'Had it been folding cards, the officials would have had to just not report the 400 cases. What are you thinking?' and 'Those who keep whining about folding cards, are you ill? Do you just want to see the world plunged into chaos??????'

In Excerpt 5, a journalist asked the commander to comment on the heated discussion online. The commander delegitimized these online comments by reframing the viewers' use of the poker-game metaphor.

Excerpt 5

1	Journalist	..網友說這個是不是有這個<MRC<F蓋牌F>的疑慮MRC>. ...想請問指揮中心怎麼看謝謝.	Online viewers asked if there is a suspicion of folding cards. (I) would like to ask how the CECC views this. Thanks.
2	Commander	...(1.3)應該是掀牌吧. ...(1.0)齁怎麼會是蓋牌呢.	It should be a showdown. How can it be folding cards?
3		把事實顯露出來就是掀牌啊. ...(1.2)齁沒有顯露出來才是蓋牌吧.	Revealing the truth is exactly a showdown. Hm only not revealing it is folding cards.
4		齁這個用詞有一點點不是很正確齁.	Hm the use of the expression is a little bit not very accurate hm.

As Excerpt 5 indicates, the journalist referenced the online viewers' use of the poker-game metaphor to suggest their suspicion of underreporting (1). To counter the suspicion, the commander reframed the poker-game metaphor as a 掀牌 'showdown,' using the deontic modal verb 應該 'should,' to characterize the classification (2). To differentiate the two metaphorical expressions, the commander made explicit the mappings between the domain of reporting COVID-19 cases and the domain of playing poker games (3). Subsequently, the commander metadiscursively problematized the metaphorical expressions involving folding cards as 不是很正確 'not very accurate' (4).

Given that metaphors highlight and hide aspects of realities, an individual can use the hidden aspects of the realities that are inconsistent with a conceptual metaphor to disprove an argument that is based on the conceptual metaphor. In Excerpt 6, the commander refuted the accounting metaphor that had been used by a legislator from the opposing party to cast doubt on the official classification.

Excerpt 6

1	Journalist	..可是剛有一個立-有立委國民黨委員陳玉珍剛才就說她覺得這個校正回歸, ..看起來像是在<MRC作帳MRC>.	But there was- was just a le- legislator of the KMT, Yu-Jen Chen, who just said that she felt the retrospective adjustment looked like cooking the books.
2		那不知道指揮中心對於委員的指教<A怎麼看謝謝A>.	Hm how does the CECC view the legislator's comment? Thanks.
3	Commander	...(1.1)欸=..這帳我們也不好作..齁. ..有病人就是有病人, ..沒病人就是沒病人.	Hm it is not easy for us to cook the books. If there are patients, there are patients. If there are no patients, there are no patients.
4		...齁這-我還是強調這對我們而言, ...每一個數目字都代表每一個病人. ..那每一個這病人就代表我們醫療的資源該怎麼使用.	Hm this- I would still like to emphasize that for us, every figure represents a patient. Hm every patient indicates how we should use our medical resources.

5	..該怎麼樣來救治這些病人. ...齁所以不是一個數目字啦齁. ...(.7)這不是新台幣這是人啦齁.	How (we) should save and cure these patients. Hm so it is not a figure hm. This is not the New Taiwanese Dollar. This is a human being hm.

Excerpt 6 shows that the journalist referenced the legislator's metaphorical expression of 作帳 'cooking the books' (1) to characterize the official classification. In response, the commander recycled the metaphor by reordering the separable verb 作帳 'cooking the books.' That is, the verb-object construction in the separable verb was transformed into the topic of 這帳 'the books' and the comment of 我們也不好作 'not easy for us to cook' to challenge the legislator's speculation (3). Subsequently, the commander turned the metaphors back on themselves for critical effect. He "humanized" numbers as people, not figures or dollars in the account books (4–5). In this sense, the commander's refutation made use of the nature of metaphor by exposing the hidden aspects of the realities that were incommensurable with the concept of accounting.

To summarize, in Excerpts 5 and 6, we observe how journalists revoiced contested views about the numerical classification of retrospective adjustment. The contestation was expressed through conceptual metaphors related to accounting and poker games. The metaphorical expressions of these concepts highlight certain realities but hide others (Lakoff & Johnson, 1980). The commander made use of this systematic nature of metaphorical thinking to refute the criticism.

Discussion

Entrenched in society is the belief that numbers are impartial means of representing realities because numbers are precise, immutable, and logical. In this chapter, I explored a different aspect of numbers by studying the semiosis of infusing numbers with judgments and values. My analysis is based on an episode during which a commander revised daily COVID-19 case numbers to more accurately represent the first large community outbreak in Taiwan. I first showed that throughout the conference, the commander used numbers talk to turn numbers into discursive objects for comment. I then uncovered the various qualities of pandemic case numbers and glimpsed the semiosis of infusing numbers with meanings through numerical classification—i.e., processes of (dis)aggregating numbers according to categorical types. I showed the unfolding of the numerical classification in narrative, graphs, gestures, and metadiscourse. The problem-solving narrative imparted positive qualities to numbers; the graph and gestures visualized numerical reasoning in relation to temporality; and the metadiscourse instantiated numerical conceptualizations of realities. The semiotic resources were used to render the invisible visible and the unknown known. Once tangible, numerical patterns and categorical relations become open to judgments and evaluations such as 那樣 ... 是沒有意義的 'that is meaningless' and 那 ... 是非常不利的 'That is ... very disadvantageous.' It is in this sense that numerical classification plays an essential role in imbuing numbers with qualitative meanings. In response to the online criticism of the classification, the commander reframed the metaphors used in the criticism, which delegitimized the accusations of underreporting case numbers.

Classifying numbers are inherently abstract. The episode investigated has at least three levels of abstraction, and the commander's unpacking of the abstraction has merits and shortcomings. The first level entailed converting an immensely complex phenomenon into numbers, which was delayed due to a backlog in administrative procedures, not testing or laboratory operating capacity, as the commander clearly stated. The second level involved sorting the numbers according to categories. However, based on the commander's talk, it was unclear as to how many days of lag would put a case into the category of retrospective adjustment. Finally, much time and effort was expended on introducing and clarifying the neologism 校正回歸 'retrospective adjustment.' The neologism is a semantic category created to codify numerical operations. Compared to categories such as gender and age, retrospective adjustment was less likely to be known by the public. Therefore, the onus was on the commander to unpack the abstract category for everyone and establish a shared definition of the category. The commander strove to do so through talk and data visualizations. Using numbers talk, he emphasized and demonstrated that there was more to the numbers than what they appeared to show. The commander also used graphs and gestures to make the category perceivable and understandable to the public.

The findings about qualitative numbers intersect with other strands of research about numbers in contextualized practices. Previous literature has indicated that numbers are powerful tools in the description, imagination, and categorization of a public health crisis (Briggs & Mantini-Briggs, 2003; Lawson, 2023). This study shows that numbers become powerful through the semiotic process that infuses them with qualitative meanings. To shape the social perception and imagination of the outbreak, the commander attempted to contextualize numbers and their associated category in the discourses of problem-solving, time travel, and contentious rebuttal.

Stafford's (2009, 2020) ethnographic study of qualitative mathematics in Taiwan suggested a number-oriented culture in which people put more faith in numbers than words. This study extends the argument to pandemic discourse by showing that both the Taiwanese's faith and lack of faith in official numbers are mediated through words. That is, before the outbreak, the officials used words to socialize the public to the belief that numbers were daily, certain, and performative in generating pandemic conditions. The belief conflicted with the numerical classification during the outbreak because through the process of retrospective adjustment, the publicized numbers became changeable and pandemic performativity, effaceable. This was because the outbreak classification emphasized retracing the conditions under which the numbers were generated. In contrast, the pre-outbreak classification stressed the here-and-now condition of presenting numbers. From this perspective, numbers before the outbreak were absolute, final bearers of realities. The gap between these two distinctive ways of numerical conceptualization swallowed some online viewers trust in official numbers. To maintain their belief in numbers as final and absolute, these viewers considered retrospective adjustment an official cover-up rather than an official attempt to maintain transparency in communication.

My analysis of this episode presents the complexities of handling inaccurate, incomplete statistics that health officials need to admit, rectify, and explain to the public. Throughout the pandemic, it was not unusual to hear accusations about policies or assumptions based on incorrect statistics (e.g., Caduff, 2020; Wallace-Wells, 2023). However, official communication that acknowledged and revised incorrect statistics was relatively unusual (see also Billig & Marinho, 2023). This is not surprising given the threat that admitting fault poses to the credibility of officials and the trustworthiness of official numbers. As such, the commander's communicative strategies for initiating and admitting statistical inaccuracies are worthy of attention. The illustrative examples of contextualizing numbers could be useful resources for creating standards regardinghow to present revised numbers to the public and what to avoid (i.e., neologisms) when explaining data revisions. The controversy over the neologism highlights the importance of clearly defining relevant categories early in the communication and articulating their significance and relevance to the public, not just to the officials responding. Although one would expect official pandemic numbers to be precise and error-free, the reality is that the numbers are used by human beings and are based on data collection methods. Indeed, pandemic numbers are prone to delays and miscounting, not to mention manipulation. Communication about repairing inaccuracies is as important as the announcement of daily case numbers. In this light, public health communication needs to be not only data-driven but more importantly, data-transparent to keep the public aware of efforts to represent volatile situations through contextualized numbers.

Implication

While the commander eloquently defended the importance of retrospective adjustment in helping public health officials understand the outbreak progression, his talk and data visualizations left the classification prone to controversy. We can draw lessons from this episode. First, technical terms should be defined in plain language and at first use (Tumpey et al., 2019). The criteria for retrospective adjustment should have been clearly defined in terms of the duration of the delays and the dates into which the backlogged cases were categorized after the delays. It was not until a day after the conference that the officials provided some of these details. The delay in providing this information allowed for conspiracies about the data revision to brew. Likewise, data visualizations are only powerful when categories in graphs are clearly delineated as soon as the graphs are presented to the public. For instance, Figure 4.3 showed the category of interpretation date on the *x*-axis, but the commander did not explain how these dates were operationalized, particularly in the wake of massive lags in reporting cases. Some journalists reported that the interpretation date was determined by adding two to three days to the testing date (e.g., Chen, 2021). The imprecision was more likely to obfuscate the outbreak than illuminate it.

Second, public attention has a limited timespan. Many online viewers focused exclusively on the announcement of daily case numbers. Public health officials need to effectively disseminate their primary messages, which in the episode investigated means effectively introducing numerical classification. Official messages that are provided later during the question-and-answer time may not travel as far as those at the beginning of the conference.

Third, public officials should avoid repeating allegations, including reframing metaphors, which dilutes the official message. The commander rejected the metaphor of 蓋牌 'folding cards' and instead proposed 掀牌 'showdown.' These metaphors became news headlines when several media outlets reported on the conference (e.g., Chang et al., 2021). As a result, the intended message of ramping up official control over the outbreak was overshadowed by the suspicion of a cover-up. Finally, classification needs to be made meaningful to the public. Transparency in presenting pandemic statistics is not sufficient. Public health officials should help the public understand what classification means at the community level. For instance, how will reclassification influence citizens' daily lives? What changes will soon take place? What preparation can the public undertake in view of these changes?

Notes

1 The Taiwan Centers for Disease Control's note on Figure 4.3: "The COVID-19 CECC (Central Epidemic Command Center) announced that it was working through the backlog cases resulting from unprocessed PCR tests. The case number would be revised after conducting examinations, receiving lab reports, and then adding new cases in the statistics. The processing of cases from the backlog, which spanned from the end of May to early June 2021, led the remained number subject to change. The community's COVID-19 outbreaks disrupted healthcare delivery, leading to the backlog situations. However, after allocating resources and enhancing service capacities, the backlog cleared in just two to three weeks."

2 While 研判日 in Figure 4.3 has the literal meaning of "interpretation date," the Taiwan Centers for Disease Control defined it as: "The date of being identified as COVID-19, which date was diagnosed and classified as COVID-19, while lab reports and clinical evidence were received."

References

Austin, J. L. (1962). *How to do things with words.* Clarendon Press.

Billig, M. (2021). Rhetorical uses of precise numbers and semi-magical round numbers in political discourse about COVID-19: Examples from the government of the United Kingdom. *Discourse & society*, *32*(5), 542–558. https://doi.org/10.1177/09579265211013115

Billig, M., & Marinho, C. (2023). Preventing the political manipulation of Covid-19 statistics: The importance of going beyond diplomatic language. *Language in Society*, *52*(5), 733–755. https://doi.org/10.1017/S0047404522000367

Bowker, G. C., & Star, S. L. (1999). *Sorting things out: Classification and its consequences*. MIT Press.

Briggs, C. L., & Mantini-Briggs, C. (2003). *Stories in the time of Cholera: Racial profiling during a medical nightmare*. University of California Press. https://doi.org/10.1525/9780520938526

Bruner, J. (1987). *Actual minds, possible worlds*. Harvard University Press.

Caduff, C. (2020). What went wrong: Corona and the world after the full stop. *Medical Anthropology Quarterly*, *34*(4), 467–487. https://doi.org/10.1111/maq.12599

Chang, M.-H., Wu, H.-Y., & Chen, C.-C. (2021, May 22). 校正回歸*400*例被質疑蓋牌陳時中：這是掀牌 [Retrospective adjustment of 400 cases was questioned as folding cards. Shih-Chung Chen: "It is a showdown"]. Central News Agency. www.cna.com.tw/news/firstnews/202105220147.aspx

Chen, C. (2021, June 11). 台灣社區流行傳播大解盲：哪些是超級傳播事件？三級警戒政策夠即時嗎？全民防疫效果如何？[Demystifying Taiwan's community transmission: What are super-spreader events? Was level 3 alert policy timely enough? How effective is epidemic prevention of whole nation?]. The Reporter. www.twreporter.org/a/covid-19-rt

Chen, W.-T. (2020, April 28). 防疫*100*天 / *120*天沒有休假 指揮中心鐵人團隊紅到國外 [100 days of pandemic prevention / 120 days without break: Command Center's iron-men team becomes famous abroad]. Central News Agency. www.cna.com.tw/news/firstnews/202004280101.aspx

Daileyview. (2022, July 24). 陳時中十大防疫金句連發！網友討論度最高的是這句話⋯⋯ [Top 10 iconic quotes about pandemic prevention by Shih-Chung Chen! This one sparked most online discussion……]. https://dailyview.tw/daily/3411

De Fina, A., & Georgakopoulou, A. (2011). *Analyzing narrative: Discourse and sociolinguistic perspectives*. Cambridge University Press. https://doi.org/10.1017/CBO9781139051255

Finnegan, M. (2020, April 8). New York state's coronavirus deaths now more than double 9/11 fatalities. *Los Angeles Times*. www.latimes.com/world-nation/story/2020-04-08/coronavirus-national-states-pandemic

Goodwin, C. (2018). *Co-Operative action*. Cambridge University Press. https://doi.org/10.1017/9781139016735

Gordon, C. (2023). *Intertextuality 2.0: Metadiscourse and meaning-making in an online community*. Oxford University Press. https://doi.org/10.1093/oso/9780197642689.001.0001

Lakoff, G., & Johnson, M. (1980). *Metaphors we live by*. University of Chicago Press.

Lawson, B. T. (2023). *The life of a number: Measurement, meaning and the media*. Bristol University Press. https://doi.org/10.46692/9781529225358

Lee, S.-H. (2024). Crisis classifications in mobility: Reporting the first COVID death in Taiwan. *Discourse Studies*, *26*(2), 242–261. https://doi.org/10.1177/14614456231219741

Mau, S., & Howe, S. (2019). *The metric society: On the quantification of the social.* Polity Press.

Ochs, E., & Capps, L. (2001). *Living narrative: Creating lives in everyday storytelling.* Harvard University Press.

Pomerantz, A. (1986). Extreme case formulations: A way of legitimizing claims. *Human studies*, *9*, 219–229. https://doi.org/10.1007/BF00148128

Stafford, C. (2009). Numbers and the natural history of imagining the self in Taiwan and China. *Ethnos 74*(1), 110–126. https://doi.org/10.1080/00141840902751238

Stafford, C. (2020). *Economic life in the real world: Logic, emotion and ethics.* Cambridge University Press. https://doi.org/10.1017/9781108673426

Tumpey, A. J., Daigle, D., & Nowak, G. (2019). Communicating during an outbreak or public health investigation. In S. A. Rasmussen & R. A. Goodman (Eds.), *The CDC field epidemiology manual* (pp. 243–260). Oxford University Press. https://doi.org/10.1093/oso/9780190933692.001.0001

van Dijk, T. A. (2018). Discourse and migration. In R. Zapata-Barrero & E. Yalaz (Eds.), *Qualitative research in European migration studies* (pp. 227–245). Springer International Publishing. https://doi.org/10.1007/978-3-319-76861-8_13

Wallace-Wells, D. (2023, January 4). 9 Pandemic Narratives We're Getting Wrong. *The New York Times.* www.nytimes.com/2023/01/04/opinion/covid-pandemic-history.html?searchResultPosition=20

Yan, H. (2020, September 22). *New York state's coronavirus deaths now more than double 9/11 fatalities.* CNN. https://edition.cnn.com/2020/09/22/health/us-coronavirus-deaths-200k/index.html

Yen, W.-T., & Kung, D.-L. (2021, June 17). 停止校正回歸、以快篩減輕採檢量能後，確診通報塞車問題解決了嗎？[After stopping retrospective adjustment and enhancing testing capacity with rapid tests, has issue of delay in reporting confirmed cases been resolved?]. The Reporter. www.twreporter.org/a/covid-19-pcr-backlog-problem

5 Classification in Mobility

In the video corpus of COVID-19 press conferences held in Taiwan, few topics appear to have consistently attracted the media's attention and required health officials' clarification over the pandemic's duration. The pandemic situation evolved quickly, and new topics often emerged, washing away previous ones. However, the purchase of the Pfizer-BioNTech COVID-19 vaccine (BNT vaccine hereafter) is a topic that stood the test of time, not because it left viewers with a positive memory but because it generated controversy and thus discussion. The controversy over the purchase was wide-ranging, involving questions about who had commercial rights to distribute the BNT vaccine in Taiwan and whether the Taiwanese government was blocking the purchase due to the vaccine's association with China. Conspirators found new fodder in the controversy for propagating their ideological beliefs. Through live-streaming and social media, disinformation and conspiracy theories spread over the public to shape their perception and thus polarize their reception of the BNT vaccine.

The controversy over the purchase of the BNT vaccine has three primary phases. In late 2020, the possibility of the vaccine purchase led to many public spectacles because the BNT vaccine was then among the most promising of the vaccines—one that could free the world from recurring lockdowns and enable the reopening of international borders. Despite recognizing the potential of the BNT vaccine, the news media fueled public skepticism by reporting that the BNT vaccine had been co-created by a Chinese pharmaceutical company and manufactured in China. This immediately caused public consternation: the idea of adopting a Chinese vaccine was unpalatable to many Taiwanese (Global Views Monthly, 2021), partly due to the transparency concerns over Chinese-manufacturing practices, and partly due to the enduring struggle with China over Taiwan's sovereignty (Davidson, 2021). The government's distancing itself from China exacerbated the BNT vaccine controversy.

One year later, the controversy still had not subsided. In 2021, Taiwan confronted its first large outbreak of community infections. During this time, the controversy over the BNT vaccine was amplified. A shortage of vaccine doses ignited public antagonism toward the government. The Taiwanese

DOI: 10.4324/9781003545002-5

government accused China of intervening in Taiwan's vaccine procurement from Germany's BioNTech (Tsai, 2021). Domestically, there was disagreement between the ruling party, the Democratic Progressive Party (DPP), and the opposition party, the Chinese Nationalist Party (KMT), regarding the import of Chinese vaccines. The KMT, which has always been China-friendly, criticized the ruling party for blocking the import of the BNT vaccine for political reasons and spreading disinformation about the vaccine (Kuomintang, 2021a). On the other hand, the DPP accused the opposition party of spreading disinformation about the government's vaccine procurement plan (Democratic Progressive Party, 2021a). Against this backdrop of domestic and international politics, health officials faced the challenge of explaining to the public the industry norms of vaccine procurement and, more importantly, their classification of the BNT vaccine as German, not Chinese.

In 2022, an election year for local governors, the BNT vaccine controversy resurfaced. This time, the controversy swirled around different accounts about how the BNT vaccine purchase had transpired and who had attempted to block it. These accounts contained murky details, fueling a conspiracy theory that the government had attempted to block the BNT vaccine due to the profitability of locally made vaccines, even though the authenticity of these claims was far from certain.

To understand the BNT vaccine controversy more fully and help advise and prepare future health officials for tackling issues that arise due to the politicization of public health communication, in this chapter, I investigate the politics of classifying the BNT vaccine as Chinese or German and the (im)mobility of the classification. I track how Taiwanese officials intervened in the classification of the BNT vaccine as Chinese even though China's Shanghai Fosun Pharma had exclusive commercial rights to distribute the BNT vaccine in Taiwan. The episode shows how officials created an association between the vaccine brand and particular political qualities linked to domestic politics and geopolitical struggles across the Taiwan Strait. I also show how, over the course of three years, government officials first wrestled with the classification of the BNT vaccine as German; then faced the conundrum of reclassifying the BNT vaccine as Chinese or German; and finally impeded the circulation of the BNT vaccine's Chinese trade name in simplified characters, 复必泰 'Fubitai,' which is associated with Chinese manufacturing. Along the way, conspiratorial accounts evolved by incorporating new details into their existing narratives. Terms such as 'disinformation' and 'conspiracy theories' were used by political parties and online commenters to politicize public health communication.

I account for the production and circulation of vaccine classifications based on three semiotic types: symbolic authority, indexical multiplicity, and iconic veracity (Briggs & Mantini-Briggs, 2016). Symbolic authority came into being through officials' use of institutional power and industry norms to quell speculation. Indexical multiplicity was seen primarily when journalists solicited and challenged officials' detailed accounts. Iconic veracity perpetuated disputes over whose account better represented the reality of the BNT vaccine purchase. These semiotic types constellate to create unique circuits of vaccine classification and offer fresh insights into contentious issues about vaccine branding in Taiwan.

At this point, an explanation of some key terms is in order. Throughout the chapter, I use vaccine branding to refer to "the process of designing, planning and communicating the name and the identity, in order to build and manage the reputation" (Anholt, 2007, p. 4). Thus, vaccine naming is a practice of vaccine branding. Additionally, my use of "conspiracy theories" follows Dentith's (2014) definition of a conspiracy, which features three components: agents, secrecy, and goals. Moreover, I translate 假訊息 or 假消息as 'disinformation' because both Chinese terms in Taiwan imply an intention to deceive, which aligns with the English term "disinformation" rather than "misinformation" (see also Maci et al., 2024 for discussions about these terms). In linguistic research, there are two primary approaches to analyzing disinformation and conspiracy theories 1) as analytical categories for understanding specific features of language use (e.g., Marko, 2022); or 2) as folk categories used by participants to associate features of discourses with stereotypical personae (e.g., Deschrijver, 2024; Tennent & Grattan, 2023). In this chapter, I integrate both approaches to examine the relationship between online comments and different political stances toward the BNT vaccine.

The chapter first fleshes out the concept of classification in mobility that is central to the analysis of the BNT vaccine episode. It then discusses Taiwan's domestic and foreign politics to contextualize the study. Subsequently, a chronological analysis of the controversy over vaccine naming elucidates the semiosis that underpinned the disparity in classifying the BNT vaccine. In the conclusion, implications for research and practice are discussed.

Classification in Mobility

Classification and mobility are interrelated. Classification needs mobility to enhance its popularity. Mobility is engineered by transforming categories in a classification system into "boundary objects" that can adapt to different social spheres, satisfy the information requirements of different social groups, and maintain consistent identities across sites (Bowker & Star, 1999, p. 16). Latour's (1986, p. 7) term "immutable mobiles" appropriately captures the qualities of consistency and mobility. Classification in mobility has consequences. For example, the classification of community spread, if circulated to other nations, can lead to the imposition of a travel ban or a change in the risk level associated with travel that is communicated to the public, thereby damaging a nation's international image and economic activities. The impact is particularly consequential for Taiwan, where the quest for international recognition is high due to Taiwan's enduring struggle with China over its sovereignty (Seilhamer, 2019).

Briggs and Mantini-Briggs (2016) theorized mobility through the lens of semiosis. Their study focused on racial and power inequalities during a mysterious epidemic that claimed the lives of indigenous children in the Delta Amacuro rainforest of eastern Venezuela from 2007 to 2008. To understand the relationship between the children's diseased bodies and the statements made about them, Briggs and Mantini-Briggs drew on Peircean triadic signification—i.e., symbol, index, and icon—and explained how these semiotic types instantiated authority, multiplicity, and authenticity in the process of mobilizing knowledge production and information circulation. Below I summarize Briggs and Mantini-Briggs's use of triadic signification to explain the complex relationships among the accounts of the epidemic offered by parents, healers, epidemiologists, health practitioners, and government officials.

Symbolic authority emerges from a relationship in which a sign and a referent are related through conventions that are independent of the contexts and identities of individuals who invoke the sign. For instance, physicians and epidemiologists ideally choose a diagnostic category that matches a disease's symptoms. Diagnosis systems often recruit institutions or infrastructure to help them exert their symbolic authority, e.g., the World Health Organization's International Classification of Diseases (WHO ICD). Symbolic authority implicates symbolic capital (Bourdieu, 1991) because drawing on symbols such as the WHO ICD requires a person to have completed special training in an institution such as a school of medicine. Therefore, symbolic authority influences the classification of some information as biomedical knowledge but other information as a conspiracy theory. Briggs and Mantini-Briggs (2016) drew on this notion to explain how indigenous parents' narratives were devalued by Venezuelan epidemiologists and government officials, who instead used medical registers to construct for themselves the personae of powerful medical and political figures in diagnosing the disease. In such a case, symbolic authority stratifies modes of knowledge production, thereby creating impediments to knowledge-sharing.

In contrast to symbolic authority, indexical multiplicity denotes a sign–referent relationship that changes according to the context or identity of sign users. Indexical meanings are multiple because they are context- and event-mediated, not conventional or law-like as in symbols. Briggs and Mantini-Briggs (2016) offered examples of how different narrative accounts and assertions were used to present the relationship between knowledge and the children's bodies in Venezuela. Different accounts and assertions were made due to different modes of perceiving the bodies, e.g., epidemiologists' laboratory tests versus parents' caretaking of their children, which suggests individuals' different proximity to the bodies. When competing accounts emerged, some were imbued with power and credibility, but others were cast as rumor, ignorance, or superstition. While Briggs and Mantini-Briggs (2016) introduced the term "indexical calibration" to explain the relationship among the narrative accounts provided by different individuals, in this chapter, I use "indexical multiplicity" to highlight qualitative differences in such accounts.

Finally, iconic transparency, or iconic authenticity, indicates that signs and their objects are related: they share at least one quality or property. That is, signs and objects are related based on their likeness. For instance, figures, numbers, and tables are different semiotic means that can be used to represent what happened during an epidemic. Iconicity also exists in texts through entextualization (Bauman & Briggs, 1990): the process by which segments of words, numbers, or figures are extracted from laboratory reports, newspapers, and press releases. These segments are subsequently woven into personal narratives or press conference announcements. For Briggs and Mantini-Briggs (2016), genre plays an important role in producing an iconic relationship between knowledge and the indigenous children's bodies because different genres code evidence in different ways and thus achieve different degrees of verisimilitude. To illustrate this argument, Briggs and Mantini-Briggs provided an example of their own challenges in the production and circulation of knowledge about the mysterious epidemic in Venezuela. They had to remove witchcraft narratives from their reports to health officials in order to avoid the reports being dismissed as reflecting superstition. To attract the attention of reporters and health officials, they needed epidemiological statements that embodied Latour's "immutable mobiles" (1986, p. 7), but they did not want the statements to be abstract and decontextualized, as this would have severed the indexical links among the bodies, narratives, and laments.

Building on Briggs and Mantini-Briggs's (2016) discussion of knowledge production and circulation, in a study (Lee, 2024), I analyzed the press conference reports of the first Taiwanese COVID-19 death across time in relation to participation frameworks. The study proposed the idea of "crisis classification in mobility" to capture the processes of making certain classifications mobile and others immobile. There are two aspects of these processes I considered: production and circulation. In regards to production, the study focused on health officials' deconstruction and reconstruction of classificatory categories through the use of metadiscourse such as referents, operators, and verbs of saying (Schiffrin, 1980). For example, health officials in Taiwan used metadiscourse to recreate categorical references (所謂的 'so-called'), to instantiate their classification principles (例如說 'for example'), and to exert their biomedical authority (專業上來講 'professionally speaking'). In regards to circulation, the study showed how classifications traveled across time and space to shape the discourse about the first Taiwanese COVID-19 death. The analytic focus was on entextualization (Bauman & Briggs, 1990): press conference participants extracted texts from a previous press conference and inserted them into another. The focus was also on footings (Goffman, 1981). Footings allowed me to study the contextualization of classifications in institutional, biomedical, and geopolitical power. The analysis illustrated why and how health crisis communication inevitably involves circulating classifications and repairing gaps in the circulation.

In this chapter, I draw on the notion of "crisis classification in mobility" (Lee, 2024) and Peircean triadic signification adapted in Briggs and Mantini-Briggs's study (2016) to untangle the complex controversy about vaccine classification in Taiwan. I trace how the controversy unfolded over three years, from 2020 to 2022, that is, from the start of the pandemic to the relaxation of strict international border controls. I also show how the focus of the controversy evolved from production (i.e., classifying the BNT vaccine as a German or Chinese vaccine) to circulation (i.e., impeding the circulation of the Chinese name of the BNT vaccine). Within each mobility process, I explore the semiosis of symbolic authority, indexical multiplicity, and iconic veracity, which contributes to the connection between classification and the vaccine. I study the signification that was used to help individuals make claims to knowledge and frame their contributions as credible or even worth repeating.

Context

International Politics

The international race to develop a COVID-19 vaccine started during the initial outbreak of the pandemic in 2020. When some vaccines were authorized by the US Food and Drug Administration for use at the end of 2020 and the start of 2021, many countries ramped up inoculation efforts with the aim of ending the pandemic quickly. During this time, vaccine nationalism also became a concern. Not only were vaccines hoarded by high-income countries, but some countries also donated vaccines to other nations as a way of projecting their global power, known as "vaccine diplomacy" (S.T. Lee, 2023).

Taiwan faced a vaccine shortage in 2021. At the time, many people rushed to have themselves inoculated due to the first major COVID-19 outbreak. However, there were not enough COVID-19 vaccine doses: many countries were competing for the then-scarce resources. Given the crisis on multiple fronts, the Taiwanese government reached out to Taiwan's allies internationally for assistance in procuring COVID-19 vaccine doses. Among these countries, Japan and the United States donated the most vaccine doses to Taiwan to help it combat the outbreak.

Vaccine donation from other countries is a significant event of nation branding that is hyped through lives-treaming. For instance, the arrival of the vaccine doses donated by other nations was live-streamed on social media and televised on the news. At these events, high-ranking Central Epidemic Command Center (CECC) officials and the representatives of vaccine donor countries stood in front of the vaccine cages for media photos. They held placards that showed Taiwan's appreciation and indicated the ties between the nations. Figure 5.1 is a photo taken at an airport by a reporter from Central News Agency. In the image taken when the Moderna vaccine donated by the United States arrived at an airport in Taiwan, the director of the American Institute in Taiwan (AIT) and the commander of the CECC pose together. Both officials hold placards that express Taiwan's appreciation for the US donation in both English and Chinese. At the bottom of each placard is a line that indicates 臺美友好 'the Taiwan-US friendship.' The AIT director points toward the national flag of the United States that is printed on the vaccine

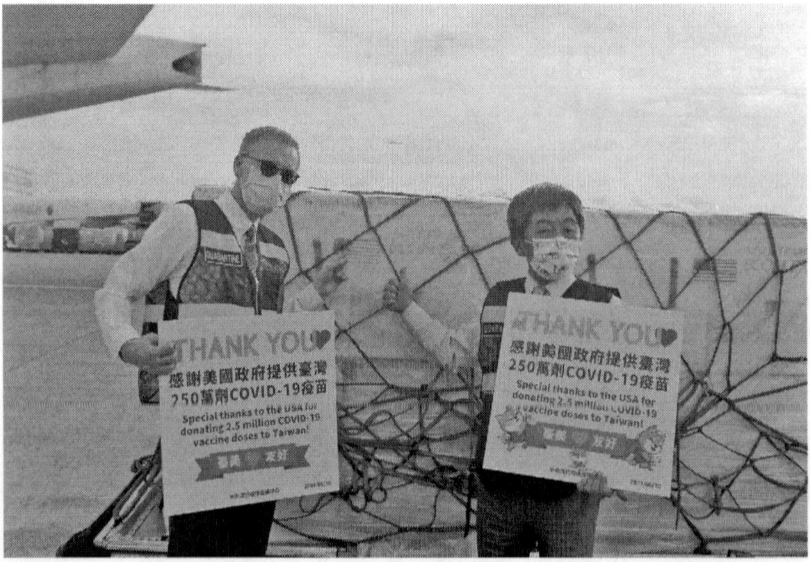
THANK YOU
感謝美國政府提供臺灣
250萬劑COVID-19疫苗
Special thanks to the USA for donating 2.5 million COVID-19 vaccine doses to Taiwan!

Figure 5.1 Government officials pose for photos when the US-donated vaccine doses arrive in Taiwan.

Source: Photo by Ruei-Chi Wu at Central News Agency and used with permission.

cages, and the CECC commander gives a thumbs-up. In this image, the COVID-19 vaccine doses are biomedical objects imbued with sociopolitical meanings via the semiotic signs printed on the cages holding the objects (the national flag of the United States) or juxtaposed with them (placards) as well as the identities of individuals who endorse the signs (the AIT director and CECC commander).

In contrast to Taiwan's efforts to emphasize its ties with Japan and the United States through vaccine donation, the exchanges between China and Taiwan about the COVID-19 vaccine were fraught with distrust and hostility. Taiwan's president accused China of meddling with Taiwan's vaccine procurement, preventing Taiwan from purchasing the COVID-19 vaccine doses from BioNTech in Germany (Tsai, 2021). Chinese officials called the accusation "fabricated out of nothing" (Yin, 2021) and offered to provide the COVID-19 vaccine doses that had been either manufactured in China or distributed by Chinese companies. Chinese officials urged the Taiwanese government not to block the import of the vaccine for political reasons. The Taiwanese government declined the offer due to concerns related to vaccine safety, efficacy, and legality.

However, the surging COVID-19 cases in Taiwan in May 2021 made the shortage of vaccine doses more urgent. Eventually, the Taiwanese government reached an agreement with three non-governmental organizations in

Taiwan—i.e., the Taiwan Semiconductor Manufacturing Company (TSMC), Foxconn/Younlin Foundation, and Tzu Chi Charity Foundation. According to the agreement, these organizations would purchase BNT vaccine doses from Shanghai Fosun Pharma, as a distributor and not a manufacturer, and donate the doses to the government under the conditions that the doses had been made by BioNTech in Germany and were shipped to Taiwan directly from Germany. This way, the Taiwanese government hoped to overcome the impasse and quell the criticism of its vaccine policies.

Domestic Politics

While the Taiwanese government accused China of interfering with their purchase of the doses of the BNT vaccine, the Taiwanese government faced accusations of 卡疫苗 'blocking the vaccine' from opposition parties. In Taiwan, there are two major political parties: the Democratic Progressive Party (DPP or the green party) and the Chinese Nationalist Party (KMT or the blue party). Each holds a different stance toward China and, by extension, Chinese vaccines.

The DPP was the ruling party throughout the pandemic. It has advocated for Taiwanese nationalism and identity, strongly opposing the 'one China' ideology upheld by the KMT in Taiwan and the Communist Party in China (Democratic Progressive Party, 2019). Given these ideological differences, the DPP has traditionally favored closer ties with democratic nations, particularly Japan and the United States. Echoing the rhetoric of the Taiwanese government, the DPP accused China of meddling in Taiwan's efforts to purchase COVID-19 vaccine doses from BioNTech in Germany (Democratic Progressive Party, 2021a). Additionally, the DPP opposed Chinese vaccine imports because Taiwanese laws forbid Chinese-made vaccines, and the majority of Taiwanese citizens distrust Chinese-made vaccines (Global Views Monthly, 2021).

Domestically, the DPP blamed the KMT for stoking fear and mistrust by spreading disinformation about locally made COVID-19 vaccines (Wen, 2021). At the height of the vaccine shortage in 2021, the DPP posted an image on its official Facebook page with the title國民黨又在製造假訊息! 'KMT is producing disinformation again' in bright yellow color (Democratic Progressive Party, 2021b). In the image, the DPP alleged that a KMT representative spread disinformation. On the representative's Facebook page, he claimed that the Vietnamese government had successfully procured 150,000,000 doses of coronavirus vaccines, which contrasted with the Taiwanese government's perceived 'slack' in vaccine purchases and accusations of 'blocking the vaccine.' The DPP clarified that the number referred to the amount of money the Vietnamese government aimed to raise from the public for vaccine purchases rather than vaccine doses.

The KMT is the largest opposition party and has traditionally been friendly toward China. However, the KMT opposes China's 'one country, two systems' policy, and the DPP's 'Taiwanese independence' manifesto because it considers both sides of the Taiwan Strait as 'one China' under the *Constitution of the Republic of China* (Kuomintang, 2021a). The KMT disagreed with the DPP government's decision to decline China's vaccine offer. During Taiwan's first COVID-19 outbreak in 2021, KMT politicians accused the government of blocking Chinese vaccines due to political ideologies and the lucrative business of Taiwan's locally developed vaccines, arguing that this cost lives. Additionally, the KMT blamed the government for obstructing vaccine purchases because several local governors affiliated with the KMT sought to self-purchase the BNT vaccine but were told that they could not do so without permission from the central government (Ouyang, 2021). As such, 'blocking the vaccine' became the KMT's key tactic for portraying the DPP as an incompetent ruling party.

Also related to the BNT vaccine is the KMT's allegation against the DPP for spreading disinformation. For example, the KMT posted an image on Facebook that contrasted a CECC official's classification of the BNT vaccine as German manufacturing with quotes from several DPP members, including the then Taiwanese president, Ing-wen Tsai, who objected to purchasing the BNT vaccine through China (Kuomintang, 2021b). At the bottom of the image is an evocative: 人民要的是疫苗 不是民進黨自產自銷假消息 'What the people want is vaccines, not the Democratic Progressive Party's self-produced and self-promoted disinformation.' The KMT also raised the following accusations regarding the government's vaccine procurement plan: 'Taiwan needs vaccines,' 'profiting Medigen [a local vaccine brand],' 'vaccine procurement in secrecy,' and 'the controversy surrounding the emergency use authorization for locally made vaccines' (Kuomintang, 2021c). These accusations emphasized the KMT's rhetoric that the government was incompetent in handling COVID-19 outbreaks.

Politicians outside the two major parties also engaged in the heated debate over COVID-19 vaccines, particularly concerning the naming practices of the BNT vaccine. A legislator from the Taiwan People's Party—which maintains a more ambiguous stance toward China by suggesting that Taiwan's relationship with China can be 'collaborative, competing, or resisting' (You 2023)—used 假消息 'disinformation' to express her position on the topic while questioning the CECC officials in parliament. The legislator later posted the video of the exchange on her Facebook to demonstrate her engagement with the issue to her constituents (Kao, 2021):

> 我們的一些民進黨相關的人士，其實大家都有截圖，你在網路上很隨性都可以看得到。他們就說呢這個我們講說，呃這個這個BNT的疫苗，上海復星的疫苗它是中國代工，中國分裝。那現在昨天莊人祥發言人也出來講說，現在這個疫苗它就是德國產製的。那請教一下，這些假消息你辦不辦？如果這些假消息你不辦，那到底為什麼指揮中心要去辦一些我們看起來並沒有真的很讓人家覺得是假消息的假消息？

'Some of our DPP-affiliated personnel, in fact, everyone has taken screenshots, (and) you can easily find them online. They (DPP-affiliated personnel) were saying that the one we called uh the BNT vaccine, Shanghai Fosun's vaccine is manufactured and repackaged in China. But now, yesterday, spokesperson Chuang Jen-Hsiang came out and said that the vaccine now is made in Germany. So, I'd like to ask, will you take action against the disinformation? If you're not going to address the disinformation, then why is the Central Epidemic Command Center taking action against other disinformation that, to us, doesn't really seem like disinformation?'

The quote shows that the legislator linked the description of the BNT vaccine—specifically its association with Chinese manufacturing and Chinese repackaging—to the social persona of green-party personnel. She then contrasted the inconsistent classifications made by health officials with those of green-party personnel. Toward the end of her remarks, she labeled this inconsistency as disinformation and questioned the CECC's operationalization of disinformation by contrasting the collective 我們 'we' with the institutional identity of 指揮中心 'the CECC.' If the CECC did not consider it as disinformation, the agency would become untrustworthy because its actions against disinformation were politically driven.

Across all political parties, the terms 假消息 or 假訊息 'disinformation' were used as metapragmatic labels (Deschrijver, 2021, 2024), primarily to highlight political stances on the naming of the BNT vaccine or vaccine-related data, rather than to genuinely engage in resolving disagreements around truth and verification. A cursory search on Google Trends shows that similar to 'disinformation,' the phrase認知作戰 'cognitive warfare' also peaked in searches in May 2021, during Taiwan's first major COVID-19 outbreak. These metapragmatic labels were often used to characterize political opponents' COVID-19 discourses, which reinforced a link between specific discourse features and an untrustworthy social persona. This persona was deemed untrustworthy because it was politically motivated and manipulated. When the veracity of a proposition was assessed mainly by who said it, a reason-based discussion became difficult. As a result, these metapragmatic labels might "hinder rather than resolve disagreements" (Deschrijver, 2021, p. 310).

These domestic and international conditions, including the metapragmatics of disinformation, gave rise to the political contentiousness surrounding the classification of the BNT vaccine as Chinese or German. To understand how the contentiousness emerged and unfolded in press conferences over time, in my analysis I focus on three aspects of vaccine classification in mobility:

1 Vaccine naming is classification because it associates qualitative categories with the vaccine.
2 Mobility entails two processes: producing circulable categories and circulating classifications.

3 Peircean triadic signification offers insights into how different individuals strive to create a credible association between their accounts and the vaccine.

Analysis

This section presents the chronology by which the BNT vaccine came to be classified as Chinese or German and the controversy over the classification. The chronology starts with production and ends with circulation. The production underscores the challenges of delineating categories associated with the BNT vaccine. The circulation highlights the controversy over the government's attempt to restrict the mobility of the BNT vaccine's Chinese trade name, Fubitai. Over time, three semiotic types—i.e., symbolic authority, indexical multiplicity, and iconic veracity—came to shape the production and circulation of vaccine categories.

In what follows, I first contextualize each press conference and then analyze the interaction between health officials and journalists. After the analysis of each press-conference sequence, online live-chat replies to the sequence are presented to show how the sequence was received by online commenters. The sequence presented in Excerpt 1 received no online replies because public attention at that time was on new COVID-19 cases.

Production

October 13, 2020. TTY Biopharm in Taiwan announced that it had obtained conditional authorization from the German firm BioNTech to negotiate with the Taiwanese government about the purchase of the BNT vaccine. This announcement, along with TTY Biopharm's subsequent failure to obtain the commercial rights from BioNTech, sparked rumors and controversy. One rumor was that the BNT vaccine was classified as Chinese because China's Shanghai Fosun Pharma had partnered with Germany's BioNTech to create the vaccine. Against this background, as shown in Excerpt 1, a journalist asked a health official to clarify the vaccine classification at a daily press conference.

Excerpt 1

1	Journalist	東洋取得德國BNT疫苗有跟中國的復星醫藥有共同合作開發. ...那=港澳台地區的這個新冠疫苗, ...這樣算不算是中國製.	TTY (Biopharm) has obtained (the commercial right of) the German BNT vaccine. The vaccine was co-developed with China's Fosun Pharma. So the COVID-19 vaccine in Hong Kong, Macau, and Taiwan, in such cases, is the (vaccine) considered to be made in China?

2		...那中央會納入公費疫苗嗎? ..這第一個問題. ...<HI那HI>第二個問題就是說,	Will the central (government) publicly fund the (adoption of the BNT) vaccine? This is the first question. Then, the second question is...
3		...如果說有跟中國..合作就不用的話, ...那有沒有其它的替代方案, ..那會不會緩不濟急. 謝謝.	If any vaccines that are co-developed with China won't be used, then are there any other alternatives? And will this fail to reflect the urgency (of the situation)? Thank you.
4	Official	...(1.0)<HI呃有關- HI>, ...這個=, <L BNT它是德國廠啦L>, ...(.7)啊呃=<A就是說A>, ...可能因為, ...中國復星因為<L有代理, ...亞洲的代理L>,	Uh regarding, this, BNT is a German company. Ah. Uh. That is, maybe because China's Fosun has the commercial right, the commercial right in Asia.
5		所以他們有..<L入股L>, 就只有佔他們股權的<MRC 0.7percent MRC>. ...夠這在, 一般=, ...<L公司的股東都有可能有從各國來的一個=股東L>.	So they have shares. (Their shares) are only 0.7 percent of equity in (BioNTech). And this in-, normally, a company's shareholders may come from various countries.

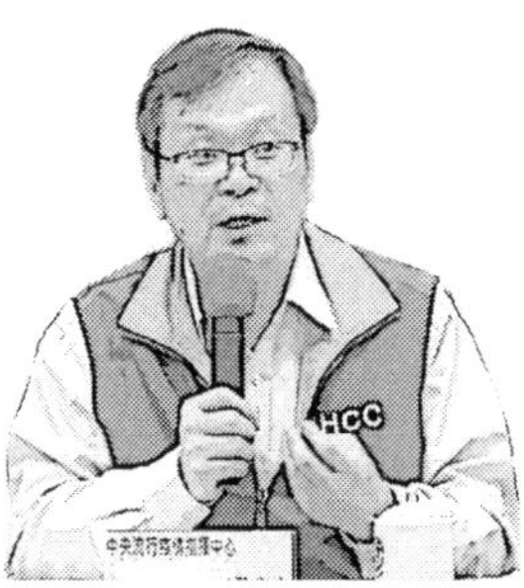

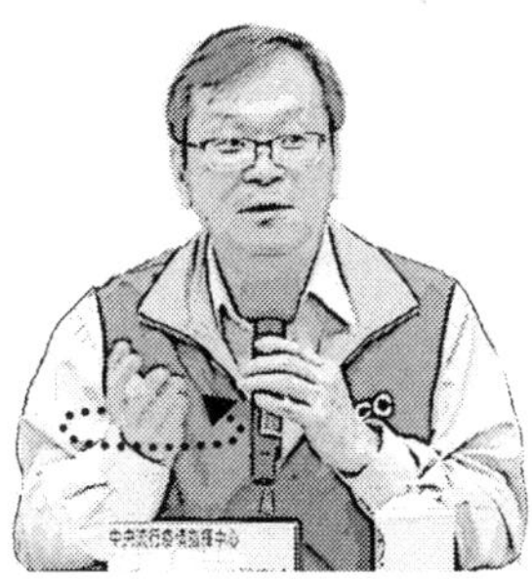

6		..所以我們不會認為它是一個=, ...中國大陸的一個=,一個廠XX,	So we would not consider it as a- a- a mainland Chinese company XX.
7		..沒有像=<A那個A>X, ...早上..揭露的好像它就是一個陸-陸-陸, ..就是中國大陸廠.	Not like- hm (what was) uncovered in the morning, like it is exactly a Chi- Chi- Chi-, exactly a mainland Chinese company.
8		..它其實是德國廠.	It is in fact a German company.

As Excerpt 1 shows, the journalist asked whether the BNT vaccine was classified as 中國製 'made in China' (1). In response, the official exerted his epistemic authority by associating the symbolic category of 德國 'German' with the BNT vaccine and offering details in quantity and quality about the relationship between China's Fosun and Germany's BioNTech to justify the classification (4–5). While elaborating on this relationship, the official appealed to the convention 一般 'normally' (5) and used the universal quantifier 都 'all' to underscore prevailing practices in the industry. Imagistically, his use of "finger bunch" (5) marked the adverb 只有 'only' as the topic of the information structure (Kendon, 2004). Furthermore, he used a palm-up open hand (5) in a rotating motion to continue the discourse about shareholders (Müller, 2004). The official subsequently rejected the classification of the BNT vaccine as a Chinese vaccine. The rejection was emphasized through the use of the institutional 我們 'we' (6), the identity match 就是 'exactly' (7), and finally, the adverb 其實 'in fact' (8) to underscore fact-telling (Wang et al., 2010).

To summarize, Excerpt 1 illustrates how classification entails producing a symbolic association that (dis)connects a sign (in this case, China or Germany) and an object (the BNT vaccine). The association was created by adopting a convention that could be applied consistently, without the influence of personal or contextual association. The official exerted his authority by claiming knowledge of the convention and determining what is factual.

May 27, 2021. Taiwan saw a quick surge in COVID-19 cases. There was a shortage of vaccine doses, and the government was under pressure to procure more vaccine doses. In the meantime, several local governors of the KMT urged the central government to open up access to Chinese-manufactured and Chinese-distributed vaccines, including the BNT vaccine known as Fubitai in Chinese and that had been distributed to Hong Kong and Macau by China's Fosun Pharma. Excerpts 2 and 3 show how a press conference became the ground for contesting indexicality as different individuals sought to (re)name the BNT vaccine.

Excerpt 2

1	Journalist	民眾ji-..關心近期的疫苗問題. ..那有幾位藍營的縣市長 要求中央開放自購的-, ...的=德國輝瑞BN..T疫苗,	People ji- are concerned about recent vaccine issues. Hm several county and city mayors from the blue party requested the central (government) to allow the self-purchase of the German Pfizer-BNT vaccine.

2		..那與..綠營立委王定宇指控, ..藍營是要進口上海復星代理的復必泰 BNT.	And this is along the same lines as the green-party legislator, Ting-Yu Wang, (who) accused the blue party of intending to import the Fubitai BNT (vaccine) which is distributed by Shanghai Fosun Pharma.
3		...那請問二者到底有何不同. ...那有人說那是中國疫苗, ..會對人體健康有影響嗎. ...這要請政院說明讓民眾瞭解.	So (journalists) would like to ask what exactly is the difference between the two? And some people said that (the Fubitai BNT vaccine) is a Chinese vaccine. Will it have an impact on human health? This would require the Executive Yuan to provide explanations for the public to understand.
4	Official	((several turns about other issues omitted))	
5		那另外就是=,呃有關=, ...這個輝瑞, ..德國輝瑞的這個=, ..呃=BNT的疫苗的部分噢, ..那它的中文名稱呃就叫=, ..噢<L復必泰L>噢.	And the other (question) is uh about hm the Pfizer- German Pfizer uh BNT vaccine uh. Hm its Chinese name uh is uh Fubitai uh.
6		...所以在香港事實上他們在施打的BNT疫苗就是, ..中文名稱就叫復必泰疫苗噢. ...那只是說是上海復星=, ...他=呃=擁有=這個=在=, ...呃香港那=臺灣這邊的一個代理權噢.	So, in fact, the BNT vaccine they are administering in Hong Kong is- The Chinese name is Fubitai uh. And it is just that Shanghai Fosun um owns uh the commercial rights uh in Hong Kong and Taiwan.
7		...所以=, ..呃=有關=-,如果是=, ..呃=, ...我們如果要買這個=, ..呃, BNT疫苗, ...噢, 那=呃可能就是=從=上海復- x-,	So uh regarding- if (it) is uh. If we are going to buy this uh the BNT vaccine uh, then uh (we) may just (buy it) from Shanghai Fo- x-
8		可能一個管道啦, ..<A就是-就是A>, ..跟BNT直接=簽約, ..噢或- 從這個=呃=呃德國進口, ..或是=, ..呃透過, 呃上海復星的代理噢. 也是從德國進口噢.	Maybe one way is- is to sign a contract directly with BNT uh or- (and) import (the vaccine) from the uh uh Germany, or uh through uh the Shanghai Fosun distributor. (The vaccine is) also imported from Germany uh.

9	...所以=呃=這個=,疫苗, ..呃=所謂的, ...<A所以這疫苗其實應該是在德國A>產製的啦齁.	So uh the vaccine- Uh so-called- So actually the vaccine should be made in Germany hm.

As Excerpt 2 shows, the journalist's question centered on different indexical meanings associated with the Chinese trade name, which required the official to perform indexical calibration to help the public understand whether the BNT vaccine was Chinese or German. As the journalist's question indicates, despite its China-friendly stance, the blue party (i.e., KMT) referred to the vaccine as the 德國輝瑞BNT疫苗 'German Pfizer-BNT vaccine' (1) and avoided calling the vaccine the 中國疫苗 'Chinese vaccine.' The KMT also included "Pfizer" when it referred to the vaccine. This naming practice was intentional. The media (Wen & Liu, 2021) uncovered that in the guidelines that had been circulated among KMT politicians, there were metacommunicative comments that advised the politicians as to how to refer to the BNT vaccine. Such comments included: 建議強調德國製疫苗 'Suggest emphasizing [BNT as] the German-made vaccine'; 建議可以統一講輝瑞疫苗，民眾比較知道是什麼， BNT大家比較不懂 'Suggest using [the term], Pfizer vaccine, consistently because the public is more familiar with it and less familiar with BNT'; and 輝瑞疫苗大多數民眾是支持的，只要強調大陸只是代理，民眾是歡迎輝瑞疫苗 'Most people support the Pfizer vaccine. As long as it's emphasized that China is just acting as an agent, people will welcome the Pfizer vaccine.' These comments illustrate that naming choices have indexical qualities, which background and foreground certain societal meanings.

Seeing the KMT's naming tactics, a green-party (i.e. DPP) legislator accused the KMT of attempting to import a Chinese-manufactured vaccine. According to the journalist, the DPP legislator used the vaccine's Chinese trade name 復必泰 'Fubitai,' which was associated with Shanghai Fosun Pharma (2). The adoption of the Chinese name and the association with Shanghai Fosun created an indexical link indicating that the BNT vaccine was a Chinese vaccine. No sooner than this link had been established were public concerns over the safety of Chinese vaccines raised (3). These concerns required official elaboration.

Following the journalist's questions, the official drew on metadiscourse to present the relationship between Pfizer and Fubitai. He used the referent of 中文名稱 'Chinese name' and the verb of saying 叫 'called' to reframe the focus on the Chinese trade name as the symbolic representation of the BNT vaccine (5–6). That is, he suggested Fubitai was the name of the BNT vaccine in Chinese, thereby sidestepping the thorny issues of indexical multiplicity (e.g., vaccine safety and Taiwan's political stance toward China) behind the naming. He then projected two ways of acquiring the BNT vaccine and stressed direct importation from Germany in both (7–8). As such, he concluded with the classification of the BNT vaccine as German (9). However, the official's explanation was not well received online. Several commenters targeted the official's use of hedges, fillers, and speech style rather than the symbolic authority of the trade name: 'Bureaucratic'; 'Evading and stuttering'; and 'Uh uh uh what the heck?'

While the health official strove to sidestep indexical multiplicity and concentrate on the classification of the BNT vaccine as German, the spokesperson for the DPP-led central government, who was hosting the conference with the health official, did not shy away from indexical multiplicity. The spokesperson intervened in the health official's speech and offered additional comments. In his comments, he imbued the category of 中國的疫苗 'Chinese vaccines' with multiple indexical meanings that reflected the stance taken by the DPP toward China and Chinese vaccines, as shown in Excerpt 3.

Excerpt 3

1	Spokesperson	中國的疫苗, ..尤其中國製造的疫苗, ...(1.2)或是他們的疫情, 噢, ..一直以來都有資訊不透明的問題存在.	There has always been an issue of a lack of transparency uh about Chinese vaccines, especially vaccines made in China, or their pandemic situation.
2		...(.7)如果直接向<L中國L>, ..來購買疫苗, ..噢恐怕會有安全性 有效性 <A乃至合法性的高度風險跟疑慮存在A>.	If (we) directly purchase vaccines from China, uh there may be significant risks and concerns related to safety, efficacy, and even legality.

As Excerpt 3 shows, the spokesperson argued that Chinese vaccines projected multiple risks and concerns. In doing so, the spokesperson conflated Chinese vaccines, vaccines made in China, and the pandemic situation into a single category that possessed the indexical meaning of lacking transparency (1). Furthermore, the spokesperson used the hypothetical condition (如果 'if') to introduce the various indexical meanings of buying vaccines from China (2).

Online viewers responded to the indexical link that the spokesperson sought to create: 'Still engaged in cognitive warfare?'; 'Changing the subject again. Everyone is talking about buying the BNT vaccine, not buying Chinese vaccines'; and 'Commercial vaccines can be politicized.' The metapragmatic labels and comments indicate that online viewers were associating the spokesperson's naming of the BNT vaccine with politics, not public health.

Collectively, Excerpts 2 and 3 show the push and pull between indexical multiplicity and symbolic authority in classifying the BNT vaccine. The health official signaled his biomedical professionalism by referencing the conventions of the industry and drawing on metadiscourse to account for the Chinese trade name. In contrast, the spokesperson who represented the ruling party seized the opportunity to indexicalize the distrust of any vaccines associated with China.

Circulation

September 2, 2021. After the ordeal of the initial vaccine purchase attempt, the three non-governmental organizations in Taiwan successfully ordered BNT vaccine doses from Shanghai Fosun Pharma. The long-awaited moment was soon to come: the cargo plane that was carrying the BNT vaccine doses from Germany would land shortly in Taiwan. At an airport in Taiwan, health and government officials were waiting for the arrival of the plane. News media were livestreaming the event. However, prior to the arrival, Shanghai Fosun posted a photo on its social media to show that on the outside of a vaccine cage, there was a banner with the characters 复必泰 'Fubitai' printed in a large font size (see the photo in Lin, 2021). Given its indexical history, the trade name Fubitai projects and assumes an image of China or of being Chinese, particularly when it is written in simplified characters, the official written language of China. Was Shanghai Fosun attempting to promote the circulation of this indexical meaning? Would the Taiwanese government allow the circulation?

When the vaccine cage was unloaded from the plane in Taiwan, the banner was missing. The absence led to media speculation about whether the government had impeded the circulation of the Chinese trade name in order to weaken the indexical link between the BNT vaccine and its distributor in China. Excerpt 4 shows that at the press conference, a journalist asked whether and, if so, why the government had ordered the removal of the banner.

Excerpt 4

1	Journalist	另外是這個今天 BNT, ...部長您也很早起去迎接. ..那在疫苗在復-, ..BNT疫苗在起飛之前說=, ..疫苗外頭是<A有這個復必泰布條的A>.	The other (question) is about the BNT (vaccine) today. Minister, you were up early to welcome (the arrival of the vaccine). Hm when the vaccine was in Fu- Before (the plane that transported) BNT vaccine took off, it was said that there was a Fubitai banner on the outside of the vaccine.

2		但是落地之後說是有人員去把它拆除. 不曉得是指揮中心有什麼樣的考量嗎?	But after (it) landed, it was said that personnel went to remove it. (I) wonder what were the considerations the command center had?
3	Commander	((several turns irrelevant to the question omitted))	
4		有關於這個齁, ..這個所謂的, ...大家有一些相片齁, 就在國外上機的時候, 齁有等等的這些宣傳的字樣.	Regarding this hm, this so-called… Everyone has some photos hm. When (the vaccine was being) loaded onto the plane abroad, hm there was some of these promotional words.
5		...那, ...探尋這個齁, 不管是台積電這邊來跟我們說, 說那個是一個, 大概是, ..BNT一向來做第一批出送的時候, ..都會掛上這所謂的宣傳的布條.	Hm, (we) inquired about this hm. Regardless- TSMC told us that- Saying that is a- probably is- when BNT sends out the first batch, they always hang this so-called promotional banner.
6		...不過跟他們的約定是不一樣. 齁就是, ...那我們是受贈單位嘛齁. 那他們是購買單位. ...齁所以他們要求就到台灣以後要移除. ..齁那也就這樣子就做了齁.	But this is different from their agreement. Hm I mean, we are the recipient unit. And they are the purchasing unit. Hm so they (TSMC) requested to remove (the banner) after (the vaccine) arrived in Taiwan. Hm so it was done in that way hm.

In Excerpt 4, the journalist requested an official account of the missing banner by carefully drawing on the verb of saying 說 'said' (1–2) without stating the source of the information. To avoid evoking the political contentiousness indexed by the trade name, the commander used metadiscourse to reframe and normalize the attachment of the banner as a commercial practice. The metadiscourse included an operator (所謂的 'so-called,' 4–5), which shows the relationship between the speculation and the official account; verbs of saying (探尋 'inquired' and 'told,' 說), which preclude official involvement in the handling of the banner; and a referent (宣傳的字樣 'promotional words,' 4), which weakens the indexical meaning of the banner as a political sign. Next, the commander referenced the agreement, which suggested the banner was invalid (6). That is, the symbolic authority of the agreement did not allow sign–object pairing; as a result, the banner was removed at the buyers' order.

The sequence was received by online viewers in different ways. Some expressed their gratitude for the donation from the three organizations: 'BNT is here. Thank you, Chairman Guo [the founder of Foxconn/Younling Foundation], TSMC, and Tzu Chi for continuing the race of acquiring the BNT vaccine.' Other viewers did not accept the commander's explanation. Rather, they considered the episode to be evidence of the government's attempt to block the BNT vaccine: 'How many days has the BNT vaccine been blocked?' Still others showed their distrust of the BNT vaccine due to the Chinese trade name, thereby echoing the stance taken by the DPP legislator and the spokesperson in Excerpts 2 and 3:

> 'Chairman Guo and Shanghai Fosun Pharma spent two months on it and finally finished making the contaminated vaccine that has the packaging printed with the Chinese characters of "Fubitai." Forced the vaccine onto the Taiwanese people. Blue and white parties, you must get the BNT Fubitai vaccine from the goodwill of the motherland [China]. Let's see if the blue and white parties live a long life, and free of side effects after they take the "Fubitai BNT." Otherwise, Chairman Guo and the blue party must be held accountable!'

Despite different reactions to the conference, both pro- and anti-government comments included conspiratorial accounts. That is, the commenters wove the information about the banner into their conspiratorial narratives. These narratives became publicly accessible through the live streaming of the press conference.

As Excerpt 5 reveals, another journalist subsequently pressed the commander to explain the indexical character of the banner.

Excerpt 5

1	Journalist	然後還有就是想要補問一下 這個, ...BNT在這個德國的這個部分 有掛上這個復必泰的..布條,	And also (I) would like to ask about this. BNT in the- in Germany (they) hung the Fubitai banner.
2		..那, ...會不會認為說這個綁上布條的話 是不是有點像是對岸在搞小動作. ..謝謝.	Then do (you) think that attaching the banner is somewhat like a petty move by the opposite side (across the Taiwan Strait)? Thank you.

3	Commander	...(1.4)沒有 我想他們有一些宣傳的動作, 那我們這邊就, ...<u>本來他們在</u>約-, 齁在購買方在約定上 就沒有這樣的一個事情,	No, I think they have some promotional practices, and on our side- Originally, in the agre- hm agreement with the purchasing party, there was no such thing.

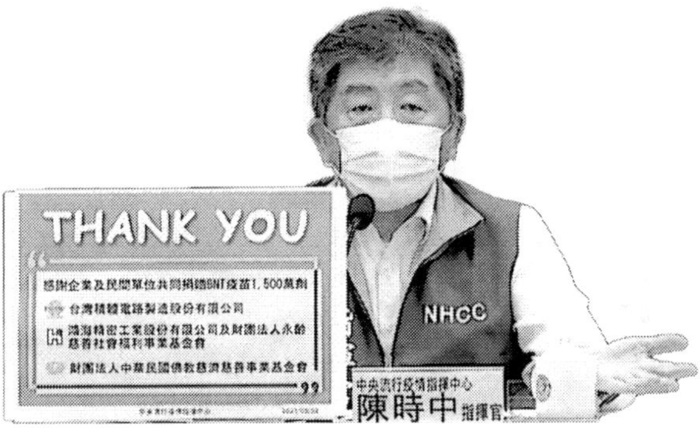
THANK YOU
感謝企業及民間單位共同捐贈BNT疫苗1,500萬劑
台灣積體電路製造股份有限公司
鴻海精密工業股份有限公司及財團法人永齡慈善社會福利事業基金會
財團法人中華民國佛教慈濟慈善事業基金會
NHCC
中央流行疫情指揮中心
陳時中指揮官

4		...那結果也沒有這樣的事情, 那這樣就一個很好的結-結果啦齁.	So, in the end, there was no such thing, and it turned out to be a good re-result, right.

Unlike the journalist in Excerpt 4 who used an open-ended question to solicit an official account, the journalist in Excerpt 5 pressed the commander to explicate the indexical meaning by using a yes-or-no question and made explicit that the banner indexed China's attempt to meddle in Taiwan's politics (2). In response, the commander rejected the indexical link between the banner and China's interference. Instead, he brought to the forefront the symbolic authority of the agreement between the buyer and seller as well as showed his perspective (i.e., agreement) on the presented object (i.e., banner) by displaying a palm-up open hand (3; Müller, 2004). The agreement did not include a provision for using the banner, thereby preventing the use of Fubitai as a sign for the vaccine. Thus, the absence of the banner was 好的結果 'a good result' (4) because it followed the agreement.

This time, many online commenters found the journalists' repeated questioning about the banner distasteful: 'Stop asking the minister how he sees it. The media keeps talking nonsense'; 'If the vaccine had not come, the media would still bring up those bad questions. Really pathetic'; and 'This question has been asked before. The journalist is incompetent.' Evidently, the commenters deemed it reprehensible when the journalists attempt to make indexical links explicit.

In addition to repeated questioning, existing and novel conspiracies about the BNT vaccine surfaced in live chat replies. One reply recycled existing conspiracies that echoed the accusations made by the KMT against the DPP government (Kuomintang, 2021a; 2021c):

> 'The dentist [referring to the CECC commander] committing malpractice, professional negligence leading to manslaughter, vaccine fraud, benefit transfer with Medigen, covering up vaccine prices, and the economic losses caused by the 3+11 policy. Aren't the Control Yuan and prosecutors going to address these issues??'

The latest news about the BNT vaccine was also woven into the existing conspiracies and accusations promoted by DPP members. The quote below shows how the demonstrative pronoun這 'this' was used to link the new information from the conference with the secrecy surrounding vaccine procurement and the DPP's accusations of China's interference in Taiwan's vaccine purchases (Democratic Progressive Party, 2021b):

> 'This batch of BNT vaccines was actually intercepted by TSMC from Turkey. Guo [the founder of Foxconn/Younling Foundation] just piggybacked on the deal, and he only issues three-month checks. Without chips, who would sell (the vaccine) to him first? No wonder Guo was complaining earlier that without the government's authorization, he wouldn't be able to buy the vaccine! If China hadn't blocked the vaccine, the BNT vaccine ordered by the central government last year would have arrived at the beginning of the year!'

These comments diverged in their reception of the conference exchanges, underscoring the argument that conspiracy theories are "ontologically subjective" (Deschrijver, 2021, p. 312).

September 12, 2022. Nearly a year had passed since the initial arrival of the BNT vaccine, and a new commander of the CECC was appointed because the former commander had entered the electoral race for the mayor of Taipei, Taiwan's capital. However, the controversy about the BNT vaccine was still reverberating at daily press conferences. This was partly due to the election of local governors. There had been speculation and accusations that the government sought to impede the procurement of the BNT vaccine. During the election year, different individuals (e.g., the blue-party and some donors of the BNT vaccine) composed new narratives to re-hype previously contentious episodes, including the episode addressing what happened to the banner when the BNT vaccine first arrived in Taiwan. Each time a new version of the narrative went viral online, health officials had to clarify why the official version was the iconic representation of the reality.

Excerpt 6 presents the new commander's attempt to stress the iconic veracity of the previous official account about what happened to the banner. During the press conference, the new commander responded to the comment by the chief executive officer of the Tzu Chi Charity Foundation, which had donated BNT vaccine doses in 2021. The executive recounted how the government would not have accepted the BNT vaccine doses had the Fubitai labeling not been removed. The new commander sought to correct the disinformation.

Excerpt 6

1	New Commander	那另外講到一件事就是<L說L>,..政府也沒有去阻擋所謂, ...有什麼中文... 復必泰..字樣這些問題齁.	And another thing to mention is that the government also did not stop the so-called- the issues about the Chinese Fubitai words hm.
2		那譬如-<A譬如說A>, ..這個曾有一批貨, ...第一批貨是復必泰的現貨, ...那它上面那個- <A疫苗上面也有這個復必泰的字樣A>, ...<P也是一樣有收件啊P>齁.	And for example- for example, hm there was a batch of goods, and the first batch in stock belonged to Fubitai. And on the- also the vaccine doses (in that batch) had the Fubitai words on them. (The vaccine doses) were accepted too, OK.

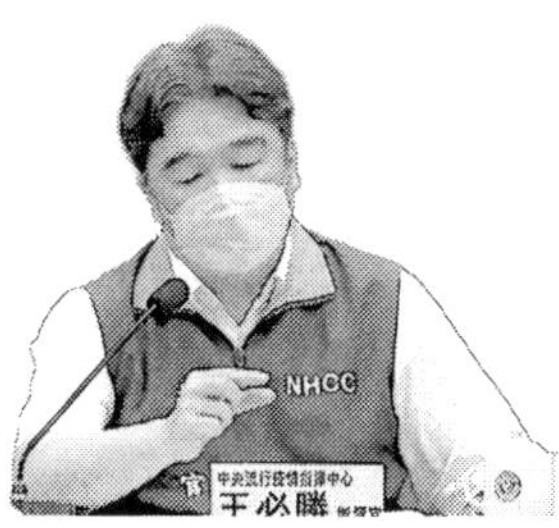

3		...(.7)那=再講到說這個=, ...(1.3)台積電那時候說, ...<L呃以跟合約不符L>, ..要求機上人員拆除這個復必泰外箱的這個宣傳布條.	Then it was mentioned again the- at that time, TSMC said uh (TSMC) requested the onboard personnel to remove the Fubitai promotional banner on the outside (of the crates) because (the banner) was not in accordance with the contract.

4	...齁那這個, ...呃並不是說=這個=, ..並沒有發生所謂慈濟的人<L上飛機..撕標籤否則政府不簽收L>這-這種事情. 並沒有這個事情啦齁.	Hm and this uh it is not- this- There was no occurrence of the so-called Tzu Chi personnel boarding the plane and tearing off labels. Otherwise, the government would not accept (the vaccine doses). This- these kinds of things. There was no such thing, OK.

As Excerpt 6 shows, the new commander amplified the authenticity of his telling through iconic gestures (2) and entextualization (3). He used iconic gestures to imagistically recreate objects, that is, the BNT vaccine doses, which in turn reconstructed the past and brought vividness to his refutation of the accusation that the government had rejected the BNT vaccine doses with Fubitai labels. He entextualized the former commander's account of the symbolic authority of the contract. The entextualization established textual iconicity and thus displayed consistency and authority in official accounts. Each of his refutations was juxtaposed with its precise accusation to directly and explicitly reject the speculation that the government had blocked the import of BNT vaccine doses.

However, the iconic likeness did not calm the controversy online, partly because the viewers were aware of the election year: 'Elections are coming, and last year's topics are hyped up again.' Online comments also diverged significantly in their content. Some commenters aligned with the KMT's narrative of blocking the vaccine, asserting, 'Use the requirements of eight major documents to block the BNT vaccine,' while others embraced the DPP's perspective, stating, 'That's right. Make it clear. It's exactly China blocking it. Now they are still blaming the Taiwanese government.' Additionally, some commenters metapragmatically characterized the online comments: 'Everyone has good intentions, so they hope to buy vaccines; but those spreading disinformation are really over-politicizing the issue, insisting on conspiracy theories.'

This flood of accusations and metapragmatic labels diluted health officials' efforts to refute accusations and address skepticism. Despite their prompt responses and presentation of key documents (i.e., contracts, timelines, and emails) intended to underscore the iconic authenticity of their accounts, the official responses were perceived as politically biased.

Discussion

Vaccine inoculation was the key to ending health emergency declarations and entering a new phase of COVID-19 disease management. While countries such as the United States faced the challenge of persuading citizens to be vaccinated, Taiwan confronted the challenge of vaccine branding. In this chapter, I have shown that naming a vaccine is central to vaccine branding, and vaccine naming inevitably involves producing and circulating vaccine classifications. In considering production, I retraced the contentious classification of the BNT vaccine as Chinese. In analyzing circulation, I zoomed in to consider the accusation that the government obstructed the import of the BNT vaccine due to the vaccine's association with China. In both processes, I argue, different individuals drew on different semiotic types to present their accounts as credible and worth repeating. Health officials relied on symbolic authority to display their expertise and knowledge of the situation. Journalists relayed speculation and accusations that evoked multiple indexical meanings associated with the naming of the BNT vaccine. In contrast to the health official's attempt to avoid indexical multiplicity, the spokesperson of the DPP government sought to classify the BNT vaccine as a Chinese vaccine and indexicalize the category of the Chinese vaccine by imbuing it with undesirable qualities. As Taiwan reopened its borders and prepared for the election of local governors in 2022, iconic authenticity emerged at the center of the debate because different narratives were competing for public attention. Their narrators all claimed to speak the truth. All political parties employed the metapragmatic label of 'disinformation' to criticize opposition parties for producing and spreading false information, citing their political bias as the underlying reason.

In the interplay of different semiotic types, online viewers became polarized in terms of accepting or rejecting official accounts. They also leveraged the accusations by the DPP and KMT to create their conspiratorial narratives regarding the vaccine procurement. Despite their differences in receiving and theorizing the official messages, the online commenters were united in expressing their antagonism toward journalists' repeated questioning. Ultimately, there was no clear winner, as the efforts to combat the pandemic were repeatedly diluted by secrecy and distrust. In Taiwan, the BNT vaccine was more than a product of biomedicine or an advancement in biomedical science. The vaccine indexed multiple sociopolitical meanings evoked by speculation, associations, and conspiracies.

This analysis thus uncovers the emergence and unfolding of indexicality, which officials can use to recognize the decisive role played by classification in shaping public perspectives and imagination. Specifically, the analysis shows that trade names are not just referential forms that attach to certain objects but are indexes that are intimately tied to the objects' contexts of production to project multiple social meanings. The case presented in this chapter suggests a complex process of indexicalization. The analysis traced the conventionalization of the indexicality, demonstrating that (1) the BNT vaccine was first issued under the trade name 德國BNT疫苗 'German BNT vaccine,' which indexed manufacturing in Germany; (2) the vaccine then acquired the Chinese trade name 复必泰 'Fubitai,' which was connected to China's Shanghai Fosun Pharma because the pharmaceutical company held exclusive commercial rights to the BNT vaccine in Taiwan; (3) because of the association with a Chinese company, some individuals started to use 中國疫苗 'Chinese vaccine' to name and classify the BNT vaccine; and (4) the classification motivated the discourse about the safety, efficacy, and legality of the BNT vaccine. In other words, the Chinese trade name ultimately became indexically evocative because it pointed toward the qualities of the BNT vaccine. Such qualities shape public sentiments about and preference for certain vaccine brands. A study (Chang et al., 2021) on online comments and surveys indicated that negative sentiments were strongly associated with the BNT vaccine in Taiwan; KMT followers were more willing to receive BNT jabs, whereas DPP supporters preferred Moderna.

Previous studies have underscored language features that shape knowledge production and circulation in times of a health crisis. Briggs and Mantini-Briggs (2016) teased apart different aspects of language use vis-à-vis symbolic authority (register), indexical multiplicity (narrative), and iconic veracity (other genres). These features and their associated semiosis explain what counts as knowledge and why certain information becomes (im)mobile. Likewise, Lee (2024) analyzed health officials' use of metadiscourse, footings, and entextualization as these officials strove to delineate the differences between two crisis categories—i.e., community infection and community spread. This chapter built on the foundation of these previous studies to explore ways of stratifying knowledge production and impeding information circulation. I hope to have expanded the previous models of analysis not only by considering semiosis and metadiscourse but also by exploring semiosis across a longitudinal timeframe and including co-speech gestures that serve various functions of classification, including marking a topic for attention, continuing a topic, creating joint attention to an object, and bringing vividness to an account. The longitudinal analysis uncovered participants' heightened reflexivity regarding semiosis, and more importantly, captured the subjective nature of conspiracy theories. These theories penetrated the live chat replies by recycling existing conspiracies or incorporating new information into the dominant conspiracies promoted by political parties. Viewing their interactions from a longitudinal and multimodal perspective helps make sense of the connection between semiotic signification and broader brand identities, political points of contention, and geopolitical struggles.

Implication

Guidelines for health crisis communication tend to focus on the ways in which officials report a health emergency to the public. As such, it is common to see guidelines regarding describing and explaining crisis situations to the public, i.e., "Acknowledge uncertainty" (Reynolds, 2007, p. 15). The findings of this chapter suggest another aspect of crisis communication that requires attention: convincing the public why and how official means will lead everyone out of the crisis. Moreover, to name a biomedical object is to classify the object according to a set of criteria and thus imbue it with different symbolic, indexical, and iconic qualities. Not everyone shares the same symbolic capital (Bourdieu, 1991) that health officials have amassed through professional training at governmental and medical institutions. As such, officials need to be judicious but intentional in naming an object that is paramount to health policy. They need to make explicit their purpose in naming. That way, the officials will actively enhance the indexical value of the name they support.

In an era in which everything is easily politicized, particularly through the use of metapragmatic labels such as disinformation and conspiracy theories, officials can depoliticize their accounts and enhance their credibility through heteroglossic voices. For example, the state government of Victoria in Australia diversified its health communication by inviting an array of individuals such as young adults, people with disabilities, and health practitioners to narrate their COVID-19 experiences and articulate their support for official vaccine campaigns (ABC Melbourne, 2021; ABC News, 2021; 7NEWS, 2021). In this manner, the officials are more likely to sidestep epistemological debates concerning the credibility of their sources.

Furthermore, officials should avoid terms that have already become metapragmatic labels in the local political context. For example, 'disinformation' and 'cognitive warfare' have been employed by all political parties in Taiwan to associate their opponents' discourses with untrustworthy social personas. Using these metapragmatic labels in public health communication may deepen political divisions rather than foster social consensus. Instead, officials should use plain and straightforward language that is free from political connotations to convey important and correct information, such as "the information is inaccurate." This approach also helps cater to social minorities who may not share the linguistic repertoires and digital literacy necessary to grasp complex crisis classifications.

Finally, vaccines need brand building to establish trust in the manufacturer and public confidence in the products. Media coverage and the positive promotion of vaccine classifications are crucial in helping the public understand vaccines (Ehrenberg-Bass Institute 2021). The findings of this chapter shows that when politics infiltrates conversations about vaccines, walking back the politicization is difficult. Nevertheless, health officials need to collaborate with a variety of experts because public health is not only about biomedicine; it is often entangled with sociopolitical and sociohistorical issues. For instance, the health official analyzed in the study could have closely collaborated with the government spokesperson or other public officials to ensure that their messaging was consistent and their focus was unified—i.e., eschewing political disagreement and prioritizing factual information about vaccines.

References

ABC Melbourne. [ABC Melbourne]. (2021, October 13). *Victoria COVID-19 update* [Video]. Facebook. www.facebook.com/abcmelbourne/videos/1010261379762461/

ABC News. [ABC News (Australia)]. (2021, August 30). *In full: Victorian health minister provides a COVID-19 update as 73 cases recorded | ABC News* [Video]. YouTube. www.youtube.com/watch?v=_nEdRT-Q4qs

Anholt, S. (2007). *Competitive identity: The new brand management for nations, cities and regions.* Palgrave Macmillan. https://doi.org/10.1057/9780230627727

Bauman, R., & Briggs, C. L. (1990). Poetics and performance as critical perspectives on language and social life. *Annual review of anthropology, 19*, 59–88. https://doi.org/10.1146/annurev.an.19.100190.000423

Bourdieu, P. (1991). *Language and symbolic power* (G. Raymond & M. Adamson, Trans.). Harvard University Press. (Original work published 1982)

Bowker, G. C., & Star, S. L. (1999). *Sorting things out: Classification and its consequences.* MIT Press.

Briggs, C. L., & Mantini-Briggs, C. (2016). *Tell me why my children died: Rabies, indigenous knowledge, and communicative justice.* Duke University Press. https://doi.org/10.1515/9780822374398

Chang, Y.-T., Tseng, H.-K., Huang, C.-W., & Lin, S.-H. (2021, June 17). 民眾因黨派立場影響疫苗廠牌偏好，不利於科學防疫 [Public preferences for vaccine brands influenced by partisan positions, detrimental to scientific fight against pandemic]. The Reporter. www.twreporter.org/a/opinion-covid-19-vaccine-politics-storm

Davidson, H. (2021, June 14). How Taiwan's struggle for Covid vaccines is inflaming tensions with China. *The Guardian.* www.theguardian.com/world/2021/jun/14/how-taiwan-struggle-for-covid-vaccines-is-inflaming-tensions-with-china

Democratic Progressive Party. (2019). *Resolutions.* www.dpp.org.tw/en/upload/download/Resolutions.pdf

Democratic Progressive Party. (2021a, June 9). 國民黨又在製造假訊息 [Kuomintang is spreading fake news again] [Image attached]. Facebook. www.facebook.com/dpptw/posts/10157650666866058/

Democratic Progressive Party. (2021b, July 15). 德國國會議員打臉國民黨 *BNT*疫苗就是中國在施壓 [A German parliamentarian debunks Kuomintang's claims, stating that the BNT vaccine issue is indeed due to the pressure from China] [Image attached]. Facebook. www.facebook.com/photo/?fbid=10157717700876058

Dentith, M. (2014). *The philosophy of conspiracy theories.* Palgrave Macmillan. https://doi.org/10.1057/9781137363169

Deschrijver, C. (2021). On the metapragmatics of 'conspiracy theory': Scepticism and epistemological debates in online conspiracy comments. *Journal of Pragmatics, 182*, 310–321. https://doi.org/10.1016/j.pragma.2021.02.010

Deschrijver, C. (2024). News media's epistemological framings of the Covid-19 'lab leak' hypothesis: A contrastive metapragmatic analysis of 'conspiracy theory.' In C. Ilie (Ed.), *Manufacturing dissent: Manipulation and counter-manipulation in times of crisis* (pp. 215–239). John Benjamins. https://doi.org/10.1075/pbns.339.07des

Ehrenberg-Bass Institute. (2021). *Branding the jab: The secret weapon to increase vaccination rates.* www.unisa.edu.au/media-centre/Releases/2021/branding-the-jab-the-secret-weapon--to-increase-vaccination-rates/

Global Views Monthly. (2021, February 23). 新冠疫苗將抵台，你打或不打？《遠見》調查：僅六成民眾願接種 [COVID-19 vaccines are arriving in Taiwan. Will you get vaccinated or not? *Global Views* survey: Only 60% of public are willing to get vaccinated]. Global Views Monthly. www.gvm.com.tw/article/77926

Goffman, E. (1981). *Forms of talk.* University of Pennsylvania Press.

Kao, H.-A. (2021, May 28). 黨團協商-上海復星*BNT*疫苗假消息到底要不要辦？*3+11*會議紀錄？[Party caucus negotiations: Should the disinformation about Shanghai Fosun's BNT vaccine be addressed? What about the 3+11 meeting record?] [Video]. Facebook. www.facebook.com/watch/?v=300372451870036

Kendon, A. (2004). *Gesture: Visible action as utterance*. Cambridge University Press. https://doi.org/10.1017/CBO9780511807572

Kuomintang. (2021a, May 27). 集體造謠！民進黨上下交相賊，全都是錯誤資訊！[Collective fabrication! Democratic Progressive Party colludes from top to bottom, spreading entirely false information]. [Image attached]. Facebook. www.facebook.com/share/p/18H7CQxA4T/

Kuomintang. (2021b). 中國國民黨政策綱領 [Policy guidelines of the Kuomintang]. www.kmt.org.tw/p/blog-page_3.html

Kuomintang. (2021c, July 20). 反黑箱，要真相！國民黨按鈴申告衛福部，涉嫌圖利高端！[Oppose secrecy, demand truth! The Kuomintang files a complaint against the Ministry of Health and Welfare, alleging profiteering in favor of Medigen!]. [Image attached]. Facebook. www.facebook.com/watch/?v=808610546516385

Latour, B. (1986). Visualization and cognition: Thinking with eyes and hands. *Knowledge and Society*, *6*, 1–40.

Lee, S.-H. (2024). Crisis classifications in mobility: Reporting the first COVID death in Taiwan. *Discourse Studies*, *26*(2), 242–261. https://doi.org/10.1177/14614456231219741

Lee, S. T. (2023). Vaccine diplomacy: Nation branding and China's COVID-19 soft power play. *Place Branding and Public Diplomacy*, *19*(1), 64–78. https://doi.org/10.1057/s41254-021-00224-4

Lin, X.-Y. (2021, September 2). 貨艙內拆「復必泰」布條恐違法？ 關務署：海關不得而知無從處分 [Is tearing down 'Fubitai' banners inside cargo hold illegal? Customs Department: Customs is unaware and unable to take action]. TTV NEWS. https://news.ttv.com.tw/news/11009020027200L

Maci, S. M., Demata, M., Seargeant, P., & McGlashan, M. (2024). The various dimensions of disinformation: An introduction. In S. M. Maci, M. Demata, M. McGlashan & P. Seargeant (Eds.), *The Routledge handbook of discourse and disinformation* (pp. 1–13). Routledge. https://doi.org/10.4324/9781003224495-1

Marko, K. (2022). Extremist language in anti-COVID-19 conspiracy discourse on Facebook. *Critical Discourse Studies*, *21*(1), 92–111. https://doi.org/10.1080/17405904.2022.2110134

Müller, C. (2004). Forms and uses of the palm up open hand: A case of a gesture family. In C. Müller & R. Posner (Eds.), *The semantics and pragmatics of everyday gestures* (pp. 233–256). Weidler.

7NEWS. [7NEWS Melbourne]. (2021, October 7). *Victoria COVID-19 update – 7 October, 2021* [Video]. Facebook. www.facebook.com/7NEWSMelbourne/videos/1019910522105297/

Ouyang, M.-P. (2021, July 15). 江啟臣籲勿擋國民黨及四縣市採購疫苗 民進黨團：須顧及防疫策略與公平性 [Johnny Chiang urges not to block Kuomintang and four counties and cities from purchasing vaccines. DPP caucus: It is necessary to consider epidemic prevention strategies and fairness]. Radio Taiwan International. www.rti.org.tw/news/view/id/2105508

Reynolds, B. (2007). *Crisis and emergency risk communication: Pandemic influenza*. https://stacks.cdc.gov/view/cdc/7037

Schiffrin, D. (1980). Meta-Talk: Organizational and evaluative brackets in discourse. *Sociological Inquiry*, *50*(3–4), 199–236. https://doi.org/10.1111/j.1475-682X.1980.tb00021.x

Seilhamer, M. F. (2019). *Gender, neoliberalism and distinction through linguistic capital: Taiwanese narratives of struggle and strategy*. Multilingual Matters. https://doi.org/10.21832/9781788923026

Tennent, E., & Grattan, F. (2023). The anatomy of a conspiracy theory in Covid-19 political commentary. *Language in Society*, *52*(4), 691–712. https://doi.org/10.1017/S0047404522000197

Tsai, I.-w. (2021, May 26). 關於疫苗，我要跟大家說明 [Regarding vaccines, I would like to explain to everyone] [Image attached]. Facebook. www.facebook.com/tsaiingwen/posts/10157494922536065

Wang, Y.-F., Tsai, P.-H., & Yang, Y.-T. (2010). Objectivity, subjectivity and intersubjectivity: Evidence from qishi ('actually') and shishishang ('in fact') in spoken Chinese. *Journal of pragmatics*, *42*(3), 705–727. https://doi.org/10.1016/j.pragma.2009.07.011

Wen, K.-H. (2021, June 23). 批藍以民調抹黑疫苗 綠：政治疫情比肺炎嚴重 [DPP criticizes KMT for using polls to smear vaccines. Green: Political epidemics are more serious than coronavirus]. Central News Agency. www.cna.com.tw/news/aipl/202106230350.aspx

Wen, K.-H., & Liu, K.-T. (2021, May 27). 網傳教戰守則 綠要江啟臣道歉藍稱網路輿情掌握 [Guidelines circulated online. Green demands Johnny Chiang to apologize, while Blue claims to understand online public opinions]. Central News Agency. www.cna.com.tw/news/firstnews/202105220147.aspx

Yin, S. (2021, February 18). 国台办：所谓大陆因素阻碍*BNT*辉瑞疫苗售台的说法完全是无中生有 [Taiwan Affairs Office: It is completely baseless to claim 'mainland factors' are hindering sale of BNT Pfizer vaccines to Taiwan]. XINHUANET. www.xinhuanet.com/politics/2021-02/18/c_1127111726.htm

You, K.-X. (2023, December 30). 柯文哲批綠可與中國合作也要對抗 藍須對抗時卻合 [Wen-Je Ko criticizes DPP for confronting China when both sides can cooperate, while KMT chooses to cooperate when it should be confronting]. Central News Agency. www.cna.com.tw/news/aipl/202312300124.aspx

6 Conclusion

What have we learned from the COVID-19 pandemic? As I write this chapter in early 2024, COVID-19 has become part of everyday life in most countries. In Taiwan, social distancing rules have been scrapped; press conferences are no longer being held to review daily case numbers; and at Taoyuan International Airport, where the first Taiwanese COVID-19 case was detected, travelers show only faint interest in free COVID-19 rapid test kits. Clearly, the COVID-19 pandemic has been relegated to history. To avoid a repeat pandemic, however, history must not be forgotten. What worked and did not work during the COVID-19 pandemic must be sorted out. How communication by turns perpetuated and eased social divides needs to be explained. Studying COVID-19 press conferences and public responses to the press conferences is a way of looking into the mirror and revealing the contours of the world's crisis preparation and response.

This book lays bare different dimensions of the multimodal classification that interpellated health officials, news journalists, and public online viewers as they made sense of various pandemic phenomena. My multimodal discourse analysis uncovered the intricacies of how health officials and journalists negotiated differences in perspective. Longitudinal tracing allowed me to document emotional fluctuations, from the desire for international recognition to frustrations over political tensions that interfered with vaccine procurement, while thematic analysis of public online responses revealed polarization in information reception and the perpetuation of conspiracy theories. Finally, in triangulating the analyses with principles of public health communication, I pinpointed some gaps between existing communication models and real-time practices in this era of live-streaming. These gaps must be repaired before another public health crisis emerges. I hope that this book has provided some ways of critically thinking about Taiwan's successes and challenges in combating COVID-19. If public health crisis management is an endeavor of mobilizing public cooperation, multimodal classification is a communication imperative in this endeavor. After all, citizens are more likely to cooperate with public health officials when they understand how the officials perceive the

DOI: 10.4324/9781003545002-6

crisis situation and why the official response represents the best-known way of leading everyone out of the crisis.

In the following pages, I synthesize the chapters by distilling the case studies' areas of commonality and variation vis-à-vis the *production*, *circulation*, and *reception* of pandemic classifications. I do so with the goal of offering ready-to-use tips for effective communication during a public health crisis. These tips can also be used to update existing principles of crisis communication before a crisis strikes.

Production

Multimodal classification offers a new way of understanding health crisis communication as a spatio-temporal segmentation of the world in order to maintain social order (Bowker & Star, 1999). This segmentation provides cultural schemes to direct official responses to and influence public perceptions of a crisis. In the case of Taiwan's COVID-19 outbreak, when public health officials did not accept the lay categories invoked by journalists, the officials drew on biomedical definitions to introduce their classifications and account for the medical condition of the first COVID-19 victim and the crisis status of the community. The introduction of these classifications emphasized official control over three critical stages of the initial outbreak. To foster family reunification, the minister of the Mainland Affairs Council drew on irrealis stories to highlight a set of criteria by which to reclassify minor children of Chinese and Taiwanese couples. In doing so, he attempted to convince the public that these children were Taiwanese, not Chinese. To correct the occasionally and inadvertently inaccurate COVID-19 statistics that they had provided, health officials introduced a new category that allowed them to account for a backlog of previously unreported cases. Because there were different perspectives on whether the BioNTech (BNT) vaccine was Chinese or German, health officials had to make clear their classificatory reasoning and evidence. These case studies illustrate the officials' intention to (re)gain control over a crisis situation, whether successful or not.

Some of the classifications the officials offered failed to garner public support, indicating problems that undermined the credibility of the classifications. As my analysis shows, among these problems, inconsistencies and contradictions posed serious threats to the official classifications. Inconsistent classifications make it challenging to know which classification is correct and which response to implement. Inconsistencies existed at multiple levels and in relation to various aspects: between government and health officials in the classification of the BNT vaccine; between the communicative modes of narrative and paradigmatic talk in the classification of minor children; and between the past and the present in the classification of previously unreported cases. Classifications also become contradictory when the classification criteria are incommensurable. For instance, the minister of the Mainland Affairs Council announced that minor children of Chinese and Taiwanese couples could enter Taiwan if they had no relatives in China to take care of the children. Still, this injunction contradicted the requirement that the children be in China on a trip to visit relatives.

Classifications are not set in stone but are subject to the volatility of external circumstances. From the very beginning of the pandemic, communication about COVID-19 showed the importance and challenges of classification. The World Health Organization (WHO) declared SARS-CoV-2 (COVID-19) a global health emergency in January 2020 and characterized it as a pandemic in March 2020. However, the WHO was criticized for acting "too cautiously and too slowly" (Sachs et al., 2022, p. 1225). Three years after the declaration of the COVID-19 pandemic, the WHO reclassified COVID-19 as not a global health emergency although the WHO reminded the public that COVID-19 continued to impact people's lives. This book highlights the volatile circumstances that Taiwanese officials encountered such that failures in clearly communicating classificatory criteria forced higher-ranking Taiwanese officials to step in and revise their colleagues' initial classifications. Additionally, Taiwanese government officials wittingly or unwittingly reclassified the BNT vaccine as Chinese, which undermined the health officials' efforts to keep politics out of the inoculation campaign. When a reclassification was made, it attracted media attention because reclassification implicated a new category to replace the previous one. However, the media was often more interested in reporting on the errors or inadequacies that triggered the changes than the volatility of the pandemic situation that prompted the change.

Of course, classification is not only about addressing seemingly insurmountable challenges. In fact, my analysis uncovered linguistic features and discursive patterns that make pandemic classification more accessible to the public. Metadiscourse played an essential role in the translation of official and lay categories. On the one hand, health journalists used metadiscourse to push for lay categories that were newsworthy: 'Why can't we just directly say an increase of 700 new cases?' and 'Is it ok to say local infection? Or is it only a case of local death?' On the other hand, health officials directed the focus to biomedical classification by annotating the categories with metadiscourse: 'We call it severe pneumonia,' 'One of its definitions is that …,' and 'The Chinese name is Fubitai.' The prevalence of metadiscourse suggests that effective communication about crisis classification needs to establish mutual agreement on the referential meaning of each category. This might explain why officials were not always able to identify inconsistencies or contradictions in their accounts. Without negotiation, the categories the officials used to characterize the situation might not have had the same referential meanings as the categories used by the public.

When journalists and officials do not see eye to eye on the classification of a crisis situation, reframing journalists' disjunctive questions enables officials to eschew journalists' polarizing categories that are newsworthy and sensational and to carve out a space for introducing classification systems that better reflect the situation. Equally important are the discursive practices of particularizing anomalous cases and grouping cases according to categories (Billig, 1985). To sort out correspondence and differences, officials must compare cases and categories. If communicated clearly, such comparison can help the public understand the intricacies of the type-token relationships in official classifications and resist conspiracies that often ascribe hidden agendas to the ways the officials classify cases.

However, in the face of a crisis, such as a novel virus, preexisting categories can become inadequate for characterizing the situation. New categories need to be introduced. This introduction can be facilitated by multimodal communication. In multimodal communication, officials may draw on gestures to facilitate the construction of new classifications. For example, Taiwanese health officials used gestures to create vector spaces, and the spaces had meanings, indicating, for example, the degree of severity of pneumonia, which helped unpack the abstractness of the classificatory criteria in speech. In addition to helping visualize the abstractness, gestures also help officials rebut journalists' propositions, as when the Central Epidemic Command Center (CECC) commander used a gesture and speech to create an irrealis case when the available statistics could not keep up with the speed of the outbreak and thus failed to represent the reality.

Scholarship on public health crisis discourse has shown the importance of metaphor and narrative in the production of official health messages. In particular, studies suggest that both metaphor and narrative may be used or abused by politicians for political gain (e.g., Hanne, 2022; Jones, 2021; Olza et al., 2021; Wodak, 2021). This book highlights the omnipresence and importance of multimodal classification in official health crisis communication. Like metaphor and narrative, classification may be politicized by politicians or sensationalized by journalists. Nevertheless, if classificatory criteria are clearly, proactively, and decisively articulated, classification can help pin down moving targets and achieve consensus. From metadiscourse to gestures, my analysis highlights different aspects of putting official and lay classifications into dialogue and making classification accessible and logical to the public. In particular, chapter 2 provides illustrative examples of effective negotiations on classifications. Only when the production of classification is well executed are the circulation and reception of classification likely to unfold effectively.

Circulation

How do classifications become circulable? To circulate classifications is to extract texts from their discursive context so that they can be inserted into a different context, which Bauman and Briggs (1990) theorized as entextualization, decontextualization, and recontextualization. During the Taiwanese COVID-19 press conferences, one way of extracting and inserting texts was to recruit heteroglossic voices and establish interdiscursivity. In each of the analytic chapters in this book, journalists were shown to be recontextualizing a third party's comments to counter official classification or to push forward newsworthy categories: 'Some people said that the Fubitai BNT vaccine is a Chinese vaccine' and 'This morning there were scholars discussing ... .' Officials also drew on third-party voices, but they did so to augment the biomedical power of their classification. For example, the medical officer drew on the WHO's definition to account for her classification of the 'severe' symptoms observed in the first Taiwanese COVID-19 case. The CECC commander and the professor of epidemiology (see also Lee, 2024) drew on the voices of biomedicine to introduce their classificatory criteria after journalists expressed dissatisfaction with the official classification.

All of these episodes indicate that circulation implicates power. Power renders some information worthy of repeating but other information inaccurate and misleading and thus subject to dismissal. In the case of Taiwan's COVID-19 outbreak, journalists relied on the representative power of the lay public and the liberty of social pundits to push forward adversarial classifications, whereas officials recruited institutional and biomedical power to elevate their classifications. In this sea of divergent classifications, the public needed a straightforward and clear explanation of why official classifications more properly characterized the situation and why other classifications were inadequate.

In addition to heteroglossic voices, placards were commonly used by officials to facilitate the mobility of important messages, including official classifications. Discourse can be fashioned into highly circulable texts that are "generically regimented, memorable, repeated forms of discourse" (Bauman, 2018, p. 14). Placards regiment speech, mold the memorable, and detach repeatable information from speech, thereby propelling information flow. Unlike the COVID-19 press conferences of other nations in which important images (i.e., curves of accumulated cases) were displayed on television screens, in Taiwan's COVID-19 press conferences, placards played an essential role in representing critical information. From reporting daily cases to announcing new pandemic policies, placards were used not just for presenting supplementary information but also, and more importantly, for extracting key messages for the public. If speech can be recontextualized to foster knowledge dissemination, so can the use of images. This is why placards at the conferences often contained figures or information in bullet points to capture the essential message that Taiwanese officials wished to deliver.

As shown in the chapter on numerical classification, the use of placards became part of officials' semiotic repertoires for the introduction of the new category called 'retrospective adjustment.' Today, in post-pandemic Taiwan, placards are default artifacts at press conferences about public health, such as the press conferences held about the mass food poisoning at Polam Kopitiam in Taipei in early 2024, because they index government officials' control over the crisis. In other words, the past is already reshaping the present and molding the future. COVID-19 press conferences have set a standard for health officials to follow or at least use as their baseline preparation for crisis mediatization.

Not all classifications are circulable. There are forces that stifle circulation. The Chinese banner identifying the BNT vaccine was removed from the vaccine shipment crate in order to impede the circulation of the classification that the vaccine was a Chinese-manufactured vaccine. Given that most Taiwanese were concerned about Chinese vaccines (Global Views Monthly, 2021) and the aim was to enhance inoculation rates and minimize vaccine hesitancy, this decision was essential. Nevertheless, online conspirators found new fodder in the incident and used it to amplify their conspiratorial accounts. Likewise, politicians who were standing for election took advantage of the incident to circulate some of the conspiratorial accounts for political gain.

For instance, the banner incident was used to reinforce the Kuomintang's (KMT) narrative of 'blocking the vaccine.' These politicians emerged as whistleblowers or lifesavers. In this sea of conspiratorial discourses, all political parties, including the ruling party, used 'disinformation' as a metapragmatic label to accuse their political opponents of manipulating the naming of the vaccine, thereby suggesting that these opponents were untrustworthy. As a result, the dominant discourse surrounding the BNT vaccine was inundated with the metapragmatics of 'disinformation,' which did not help resolve disagreements.

Each time a new conspiratorial account about the BNT vaccine went viral online, health officials at the press conferences were forced to clarify that the banner had been removed due to contractual requirements, not political motives. Despite the officials' efforts and quick responses, public perceptions of the BNT vaccine were heavily skewed by political preferences, not by public health officials' professional advice. The banner incident is a resounding example of how public health crisis communication can be politicized through classification in (im)mobility and the metapragmatics of 'disinformation.' When politics intrudes on public health communication, discourses about the crisis come into conflict, and collaboration across social scales is stifled.

Why do some classifications travel broadly but others are prone to distortion and resistance? Constructing classifications that are mobile and continuous, which Latour (1986) called "immutable mobiles," is more complex than how it is described in the Taiwanese communication guidelines: "Make use of various approaches" and "Strengthen communication with the media" (Taiwan Centers for Disease Control, 2020, p. 9–10). There are two challenges to overcome when making a classification circulable without sacrificing its precision. First, circulation is subject to pre-existing social fractures. The pandemic exacerbated social divides that had existed even before the pandemic. In Taiwan, distrust of China had reached new heights following protests in Hong Kong against the introduction of controversial extradition laws, as well as the presidential election in Taiwan in January 2020, which had fueled heated discussions about the sovereignty of Taiwan. As such, when the pandemic hit, any categories associated with China became targets for politicization. The naming of the BNT vaccine exemplifies the politicization of classification. Second, central to circulation is the practice of extracting and inserting categories in different contexts. Biomedical classification allows for few changes and little improvisation because not everyone has the epistemology for making these changes. In contrast, classification that is not biomedicine-related is more likely to be reinterpreted, as in the classification of Xiao Ming.

To summarize, circulating classifications widely and proactively is a key determinant of successful crisis responses. Impeding inaccurate classification is equally important in the shaping of public perspectives. Effective circulation also needs to consider the uptake of these circulatory processes, which is also known as reception or consumption.

Reception

My analysis of Taiwan's COVID-19 press conferences highlights that live-streaming can bring fundamental changes to how health messages are received. Journalists were no longer the only audience for press conferences. Health officials also spoke directly to the public by live-streaming the conferences on social media platforms such as Facebook and YouTube. Rather than serving as passive receivers of official classifications, public online viewers could comment on the classifications through the functions of "add comment" and "live chat." Thus, the widespread adoption of live-streaming technology can contribute to public participation in and consumption of health crisis communication because live-streaming replaces one-way information transmission with more direct two-way exchanges between officials and communities. However, live-streaming also poses new challenges.

Live-streaming may polarize online participation. Public online commenters offered panoptical assessments of the interactions between journalists and officials, especially when the officials and journalists disagreed on which categories to use and whose classification was more suitable. The assessments were made by two primary groups of online commenters: pro-government followers and anti-government problematizers. The problematizers questioned many aspects of the official communication. Their critical assessment of the communication revealed their ideological beliefs about how health crisis communication should or should not be conducted. The ideologies ranged from prosody, 'Evading and stuttering'; to neologism, 'Shih-Chung Chen, the term inventor'; topic, 'Changing the subject again. Everyone is talking about buying the BNT vaccine, not buying Chinese vaccines'; and finally, to speech genre, 'What ghost story are you fabricating?' In contrast, online followers who supported the official account engaged in the discussion by attacking those who held different viewpoints: 'Go back to school, OK? The term already exists' and 'Those (people) who are still asking about retrospective adjustment. Are they illiterate?' As a result, what was meant to be a digital space for engaging the public became a forum for airing polarized views about an issue. Sun's (2023) quantitative analysis of live-chat replies indicated that the polarization was more severe after the first outbreak in Taiwan in 2021 than it was during the 2020 outbreaks worldwide. Such splits in public opinion can hinder collaboration and discourage other individuals from participating in the discussion. As such, online live-chat replies may perpetuate self-validation and the polarization of existing beliefs rather than engagement with diverse views and values (Harel et al., 2020).

Live-streaming may also make it more difficult to tackle conspiratorial discourses and thus reach public consensus on classification. Online commenters, be they pro-government followers or anti-government problematizers, interpreted official messages as new evidence of secrecy, thereby reinforcing their own conspiratorial accounts. The chapter about the naming practice of the BNT vaccine addresses this issue. The online commenters who subscribed to the KMT's narrative of 'blocking the vaccine' considered the removal of the banner on the crate housing the BNT vaccine to be part of the government's conspiracy to block the vaccine. Meanwhile, the commenters who supported the DPP's classification of the BNT vaccine as Chinese adapted the banner incident to fit their accounts of collusion between China and KMT affiliates. These accounts can be considered conspiratorial because they feature the three necessary elements of conspiracy: plotters, secrecy, and goals (Dentith, 2014, p. 23). These examples of the BNT vaccine's reception illustrate how new information can be easily incorporated into conspiracy theories and ultimately influence the public reception of an event. Tackling these conspiratorial discourses is challenging because live-streaming allows individuals to engage anonymously in public health communication.

Moreover, recent research in discourse analysis has highlighted the importance of understanding the pandemic term "conspiracy theory" as a metapragmatic label (Deschrijver, 2024) or social action (Tennent & Grattan, 2023), because the term can be used or recognized by different individuals to reflect their ideas about language use in particular contexts. This is indeed the case in the live-chat replies to the press conference videos. Online commenters not only shared their thoughts, but they also indicated their stance toward other commenters' comments. In such cases, terms such as 'conspiracy theory' and 'cognitive warfare' often became metapragmatic labels for characterizing other viewers' discourses as false and misleading. The characterization created social divisions rather than facilitating meaningful engagement in discussions about public health.

Live-streaming exposes the processes of producing newsworthy information, thereby positioning journalists as 'co-performers' in a live show (Wei, 2020). As a result, journalists' strategies for soliciting newsworthy information are scrutinized, assessed, and even criticized by public online commenters. For instance, repeated questioning is a strategy commonly used by journalists to press interviewees to answer questions directly and disclose further details (Chang, 2021). However, in the case of Taiwan's COVID-19 outbreak, the strategy often triggered sharp criticism from online commenters who were pro-government followers: 'This question has been asked before. The journalist is incompetent'; 'If there is no question, stop seeking attention. Journalist'; and 'Not yet. The journalist can't understand it.' This hostile stance toward journalistic questions was a double-edged sword (Chang, 2021). In some cases, the journalists became more conscious of their tone and diction in framing the questions; they also made explicit the importance and relevance of their questions to the public concerns. In other cases, journalists began to practice self-censorship by reconsidering those questions that sought to hold officials accountable for their decisions. Some even abandoned opportunities to question or pursue officials altogether.

Live-streaming makes official classification public and transparent, as shown during Taiwan's COVID-19 outbreak when Taiwanese health officials remained at almost all the press conferences until all journalists' questions had been answered. Nevertheless, speaking turns at the conferences were strictly controlled by the officials, allowing them to exert some control over how their responses were received. As an example, consider the question-and-answer session held during each conference. Each session was conducted such that journalists had to bid for the CECC commander's permission to speak. Upon being selected to speak, a journalist had to ask all of their questions at once, and the officials answered all the questions before taking questions from other journalists. In other words, the journalist who had been selected by the commander could not immediately take a second turn following up on the official response. The one-turn-per-time norm forced the journalist to accept whatever answers the officials provided. While the journalist could rely on fellow journalists to ask follow-up questions, the journalists were not always interested in the same topics. By exerting control over speaking turns, the officials forced journalists to surrender their power of pressing the officials for critical information that concerned the public (Chang, 2021).

Still, some journalists were not shy in voicing their dissatisfaction with officials' evasions and dismissals. They directly criticized the officials for their muddled classification, 'What you just said is a com- complete contradiction of yourself,' and demanded straightforward classification, 'If yes, just say yes. If no, just say no.' Some journalists adopted the more indirect tactic of assuming the role of an animator (Goffman, 1981) who relayed criticism from others to characterize the official classification: 'Online viewers asked if there is a suspicion of folding cards. I would like to ask how the CECC views this' and 'But there was- was just a le- legislator of the KMT, Yu-Jen Chen, who just said that she felt the retrospective adjustment looked like cooking the books.' In adopting these strategies, the journalists revealed their ideological belief that the role of media is to hold the government accountable for its policies and decisions.

In summary, live-streaming empowers health officials to directly engage the public in the reception and consumption of public health messages. However, live-streaming also poses new challenges for journalists in facilitating the public uptake of pandemic information. The public can receive and respond to official health communication more easily and directly than ever before, but their varied reception of official information becomes evident, which in turn undercuts the possibility of collaboration in times of crisis. When live-streaming becomes the predominant mode of communication in crises, further research is required on how to better engage journalists, rather than sidelining their participation or vilifying them for holding officials accountable. Equally necessary is a fuller understanding of how to turn public online spaces into forums for effective engagement and meaningful discussion, not spaces for perpetuating conspiracies and spreading false information.

Towards Effective Crisis Communication in Public Health

For health crisis communication to be effective, it needs to be revised and updated according to evolving trends in communication and advancements in technology. The advent of live-streaming and the widespread use of multimodality led to fundamental changes in Taiwanese health crisis communication. These changes came with new challenges. I have uncovered some of the challenges in the analytical chapters. Below, I offer five suggestions for making principles of public health communication more up-to-date and inclusive. The suggestions are based on my multimodal analysis of Taiwanese officials' classification practices, existing literature on multimodal discourse analysis (e.g., Lempert, 2011; McNeill, 2005), and various sets of crisis communication guidelines (e.g., Reynolds, 2007; Taiwan Centers for Disease Control, 2020; Tumpey et al., 2019;). The suggestions are not meant to replace existing principles but to nuance them. In offering these suggestions, I contribute to discussions on how to make public health information more accessible to broader audiences, particularly social minorities.

Expand Multimodal Use

Expand the definition of multimodality so that it reaches beyond the use of multiple channels (i.e., television broadcasts and social media live-streaming). Learning how to navigate multimodal repertoires is crucial for health officials and requires practice. However, to help expedite the learning process, I have compiled a taxonomy of the multimodal repertoires used in the conference sequences analyzed in this book. Table 6.1 presents this taxonomy of multimodal types and features and provides examples from Taiwan's COVID-19 crisis classification experience. The taxonomy ranges from gestures, hand motions, corporeal orientation, material artifacts, and finally, to participation frameworks. The use of more multimodalities needs to be coordinated with a clear and consistent explanation of classification criteria and categorical definitions. That is, speech and multimodalities must be treated as inseparable in presenting health crisis information.

Make Health Messages Circulable

In a sea of information, the public is keen to know which information is important, why it matters to them, and what they can do to prepare for any impending changes. Officials who strive to promote effective public health communication should proactively put key public health messages into circulation rather than passively waiting for journalists to filter newsworthy information to the public. There are three tips officials can follow to support effective circulation.

Table 6.1 Taxonomy of multimodal repertoires

Type	*Feature*	*Example*
Iconic gesture	An iconic gesture creates an image of a concrete object or action. The image resembles the description of an event in speech; the resemblance helps the public understand which aspects of the object or action the speaker is focusing on. Use an iconic gesture when you are providing concrete examples to elaborate on an argument; an iconic gesture can make the elaboration more vivid and accessible.	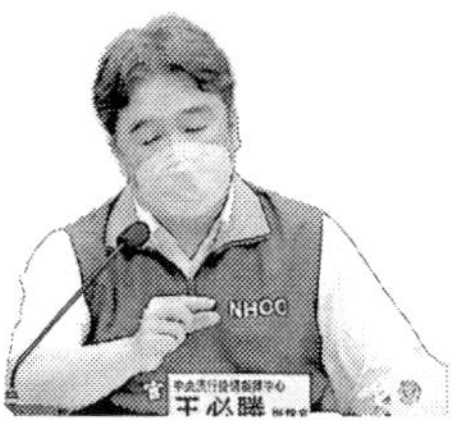 那它上面那個- 疫苗上面也有這個復必泰的字樣 'And on the- also the vaccine doses had the Fubitai words on them.'
Metaphoric gesture	A metaphoric gesture is an image of the abstract. The abstract meaning can exist in the speaker's hand shape or space. Use a metaphoric gesture to unpack abstract concepts for the public. A metaphoric gesture is best combined with real-life examples to establish a common understanding. Ensure the examples and the metaphoric gesture are consistent and coherent.	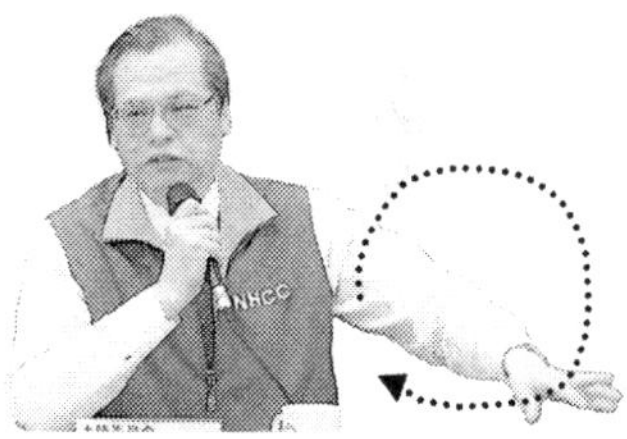 陸配的大陸親人 'mainland spouses' mainland relatives'
Palm-up open hand	A palm-up open hand is a type of metaphoric gesture. When a speaker uses a palm-up open hand, they appear to be holding an object. It is as if they are presenting an idea in their hand for scrutiny. This type of gesture has multiple communication functions, including engaging the audience, asserting authority, and continuing a topic.	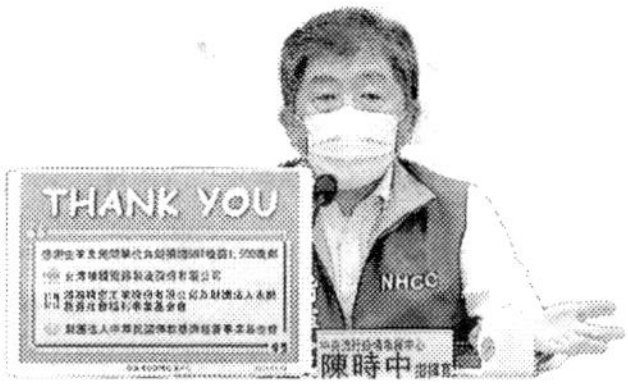 本來他們在約-, 齁在購買方在約定上'Originally, in the agre- hm agreement with the purchasing party,'
Precision-Grip gesture	A precision grip is created when the speaker connects their thumb to the tip of their forefinger. A precision grip has a focus-on effect in communication and should only be used to make sharp, effective points. Before communicating, think about what the most important message is and then use a precision grip to help the audience identify the key message in the speech.	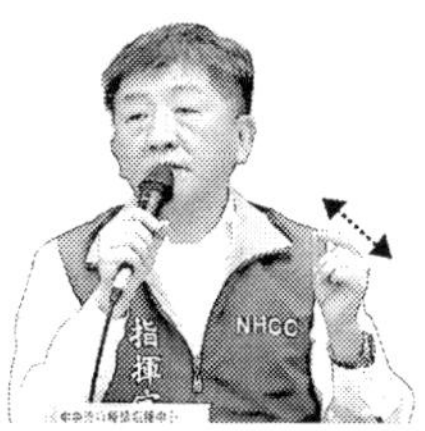 通常齁它有幾樣的徵兆，齁專業上來講 'usually mh it has several kinds of signs, mh professionally speaking.'

(*Continued*)

Table 6.1 (Continued)

Type	*Feature*	*Example*
Gesture vector	A gesture vector translates an abstract concept into a visual representation. The gesture space exemplifies the degree of a specific quality, such as the transmission rate or severity of a disease. Use a gesture vector to make a concept accessible to your audience. For example, when a new category is introduced to account for present circumstances, you can use a gesture vector to help establish a common understanding.	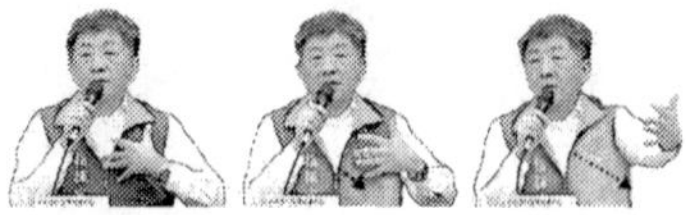 一傳十十傳百 'One spreads to ten. Ten spread to one hundred.'
Irrealis gesture	An irrealis gesture aids in explaining hypothetical situations. This gesture can be a useful way of problematizing inaccurate speculations or exhorting the public to follow official orders. Use hypothetical reasoning and an irrealis gesture only when they help clarify why a proposed change is important. Otherwise, emphasize facts; explain what you already know and what you plan to do.	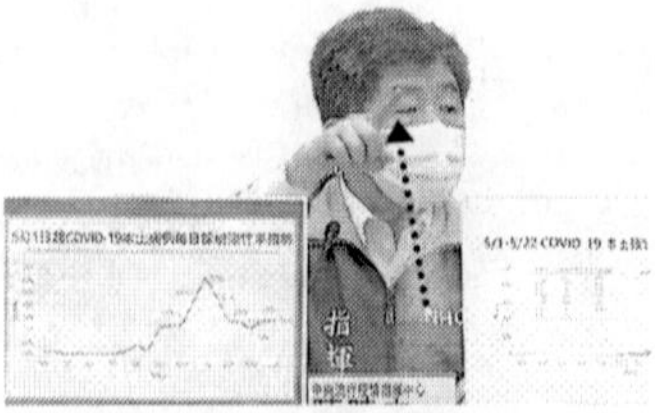 那你會造成很大的一個誤解. 'you would then bring about a very big misinterpretation.'
Placard	A placard is a visual board that can be carried to a press conference and mounted on the table with a holder. Use a placard to visualize categorical relationships and summarize key public health information. Circulate the electronic version of the placard online and with journalists to reinforce the reception of the information. Avoid providing details in a placard; instead include QR codes for the public to find more information.	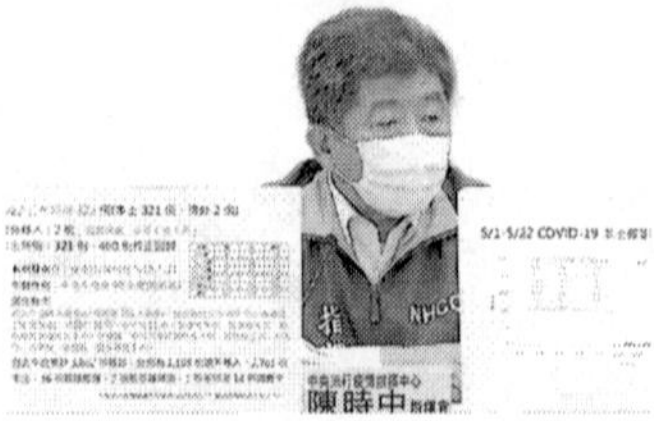

Table 6.1 (Continued)

Type	*Feature*	*Example*
Symbolic object	Objects at press conferences, particularly those positioned in front of the camera, attract attention because they may symbolize certain values, beliefs, or ideologies. Use symbolic objects strategically. Objects' shapes and colors also express meanings. Be aware of the meanings objects express. The strategic use of objects can generate media coverage and garner public attention. Overly relying on objects to maintain public interest, however, can detract from key messaging.	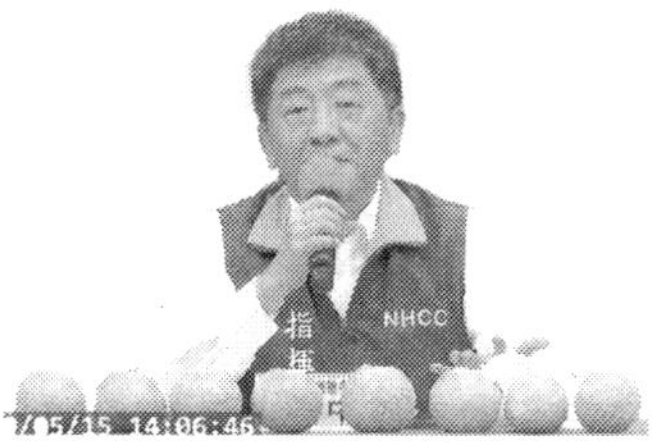
Corporeal orientation	Corporeal orientation refers to the use of body in relation to others. Be cautious with your body language. Changes in body orientation express meanings. If you are sitting on a panel and facing reporters, your gaze and body movement toward other panelists can indicate whether you (dis)agree with what they are saying.	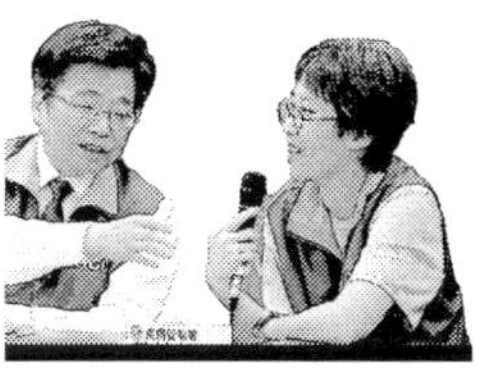
Participation framework	The participation framework refers to ways of engaging in press conferences, including seating arrangements and turn-taking norms of speaking. Present yourself as on a team with your colleagues during conferences; speak as a team, for example, by using the collective pronoun of "we" or an institutional reference such as "Central Epidemic Command Center." All key players should face the media. Introduce each official and identify their subject-matter expertise. The image of a unified team conveys a sense of well-preparedness and a concerted effort to bring the crisis under control. Appoint a moderator to allocate speaking turns. Live-stream not just speakers' facial expressions but also their use of objects and body language.	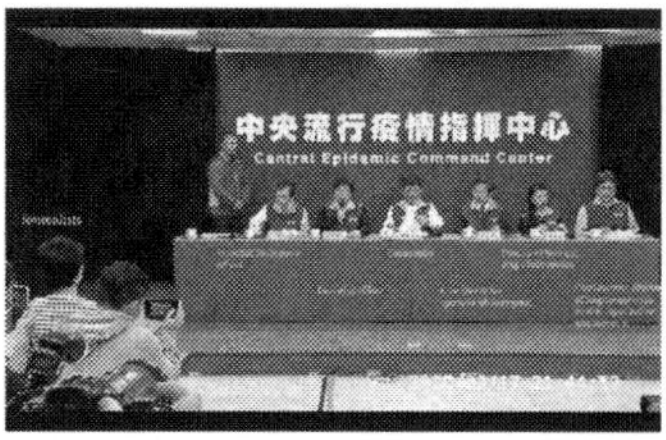

First, make key public health messages *easy to repeat.* Start with identifying key categories that need to be spread broadly and quickly. A useful method is to consider which categories you would like to see in the news headlines reporting on the conference. After identifying the categories, practice explaining them in plain language and with everyday examples. Avoid acronyms and technical terms that are difficult to say or remember. Use multimodalities such as placards because they make the categories and explanations easy to extract.

Second, make the messages *worth repeating.* Explain the impact that the crisis will have on the public. Avoid exaggerating the impact or speculating on the worst-case scenario. Instead, help the public develop reasonable expectations. Avoid dichotomizing people as either in-group or out-group, as doing so marginalizes and, at worst, vilifies certain populations. Instead, be inclusive. Focus on the impact on all individuals and appeal to collective responsibility.

Finally, make the message *practical for repeating.* Connect the message with specific actions that people can take to prepare for the change. That way, they feel more in control of the situation and are more likely to engage others. A strong connection between action and message is indicated by people engaging in the same action and sharing an understanding of the key message.

Minimize Gaps in Classifications

Much communicative controversy stems from gaps in classifications in official communication, whether the gaps originate across government departments or between central and local governments. Moving forward, health officials need to establish guidelines on how to effectively classify various phenomena related to public health crises. Such guidelines could start with default classifications that inevitably require clarification, such as "restriction orders" and the "three first times": the first confirmed case, the first community-infection case, and the first death. Subsequently, the focus can be extended to include more localized classifications, such as "Chinese vaccines," which require an understanding of biomedical legality and industry norms. Although gaps are inevitable among officials, journalists, and the public, these guidelines can help officials proactively repair them: for example, by juxtaposing different interpretations and pointing out the reasoning behind the official classification and the fallacies in the alternative classifications. Changing classificatory definitions after they are made public generates controversy rather than repairing gaps. Therefore, official classifications need to be created according to clearly stated principles.

Tackle Classification Questions Effectively

Public health crisis communication inevitably requires officials to present and explain their classifications of crisis phenomena. Journalists commonly ask for clarification on classificatory criteria, the definitions of categories, and official responses to disagreements by media or political pundits. Therefore, officials must be very aware of the types of classifications before they can provide effective responses. Table 6.2 shows five types of classification questions typically asked by journalists. The question types are not mutually exclusive. For example, a speculative question may also be a metadiscourse question. However, each question type emphasizes different aspects of classification: language use (metadiscourse), forcefulness and newsworthiness (disjunctive), affective speculation (speculation), disagreement (third party), and the extension from the known to the unknown (inference).

After identifying classification questions and their focus, officials can use Table 6.3 to formulate an effective response to each question. The strategies and examples in Table 6.3 are organized according to discourse moves. After receiving a question, first, restate it. Restate the question to establish common ground before launching into a response. Restating a question is especially important when journalists ask several different questions at once. Take the opportunity to reframe the question in a way that more people can understand the focus of the question easily. If an official classification has already been determined, respond directly and firmly. Avoid noun phrases that have been politicized in the local context, such as 'disinformation' in Taiwan. If a classification has yet to be made,

Table 6.2 Types of journalists' questions about classification

Metadiscourse: Seek clarification on language choices. Metadiscourse usually occurs when a category is technical or there is a gap between lay and professional understandings of the category.

• 那想問這個400例的回歸是不是全-..世界,..台灣首創的名詞謝謝.

'Hm I would like to ask if the 400 cases of retrospective (adjustment)- Is Taiwan the first in the whole- world to initiate the use of this term? Thanks.'

Disjunctive: Push officials to directly answer questions and identify newsworthy categories. Because these dual functions serve well the purpose of journalism, the disjunctive format is commonly used by journalists.

• 那名台商是重症還是輕症, 從臨床判斷.

'Are the Taiwanese businessperson's symptoms severe or mild, clinically diagnosed?'

Speculation: Speculate on motives behind a classification. Speculative questions can easily propel conspiracy theories, but they also offer opportunities for officials to rebut the theories.

• 今天我們增加回歸的這400例,...就大家還是蠻疑惑的, 為什麼我們就不直接講說就是新增700是擔心大家會-... 因為聽到這個數字而嚇到嗎.

'Today we have 400 cases of retrospective adjustment. Everyone is still quite confused. Why can't we just directly say it is a new addition of 700 cases? Is it because of the worry that everyone will be scared when hearing the number?'

Third party: Seek official responses to disagreements, inconsistencies, or criticisms. The third-party question type is the most confrontational type.

• 可是剛有一個立-有立委國民黨委員陳玉珍剛才就說她覺得這個校正回歸, 看起來像是在作帳. 那不知道指揮中心對於委員的指教怎麼看謝謝.

'But there was- was just a le- legislator of the KMT, Yu-Jen Chen, who just said that she felt the retrospective adjustment looked like cooking the books. Hm how does the CECC view the legislator's comment? Thanks.'

Inference: Use what is known to arrive at a classification and seek official confirmation.

• 所以我們這樣會研判說中國境內已經有社區感染的病狀

'So we can judge that there are already signs of community infection in China?'

Table 6.3 Response strategies and examples

- *Restate and reframe the question*: Establish a shared understanding of the question before responding. Make the question understandable to broader audiences.

好這個病例為什麼要回歸啦齁.

'OK why did we retrospectively adjust the numbers?'

- *Respond directly and with certainty*: State what the classification is and is not before providing an explanation. Use the structure of 是A (而)不是B 'it is A rather than B' to emphasize the contrast between correct and incorrect classifications.

今天被確診, 她就是我們所謂的嚴重肺炎... 齁所以不是在嚴重肺炎裡面的重症

'Today having been confirmed as a COVID-19 case, she is the so-called having severe pneumonia … Okay so it is not the severe symptom in severe pneumonia.'

- *Admit the unknown and share the known*: It is okay not to have an immediate answer to a journalist's question. But state what you do know.

不太清楚其他國家的那個國籍嘿... 嘿因為泰國的話他們是

'Not clear about the nationalities of other countries' cases, mh... Mh because in the case of Thailand, they are....'

- *List criteria*: Use signal words to guide the public if there is more than one criterion to consider.

一個是... 然後第二個是... 然後第三個... 然後第四個是說...

'One is ... Then the second one is ... Then the third one ... Then the fourth one is ... .'

- *Apply each criterion immediately*: As soon as a criterion is introduced, use the criterion to classify the crisis. Do not wait until all criteria are introduced to classify the crisis.

一個是確定病例無法找出感染來源. 就跟我們今天,目前的情況是一樣的

'One is being unable to find the infection source of a confirmed case. Just like us today. The current situation is the same.'

- *Enhance credibility*: Recruit subject-matter experts to endorse the classification and depoliticize the topic. Make each expert's identity and expertise known to the audience.

請問那個-路-這路徑齁是不是要讓張教授來補充

'Ask the- path- the pathway mh. Should we ask Professor Zhang to supplement information?'

- *Reiterate classification*: Repeat official classification at the end to leave a strong impression on the audience. Preface the reiteration with discourse connectives, for example, 所以 'so.'

所以我們不會認為它是一個=,...中國大陸的一個=,一個廠XX … 它其實是德國廠

'So we would not consider it as a- a- a mainland Chinese company XX. It is in fact a German company.'

be frank and admit the unknown. Then provide the public with what you do know. At times, you may need to convince the public by working through a list of classificatory criteria. Each time you explain a criterion, apply the criterion to the crisis and tell everyone whether the crisis situation meets the criterion. Additionally, consider recruiting subject-matter experts to enhance the credibility of the classification and depoliticize the topic. Before concluding your response, push the official classification further by reiterating the categories. Together, these strategies will help you put the crisis in proper perspective.

Translate Classification into Meaningful Categories

Not all categories of classification are easily understandable by the public. Some categories have different meanings in biomedicine and everyday use. Metadiscourse can help bridge the biomedical world and the everyday world. Before making official classifications public or responding to journalists' questions about classifications, carefully think through the categories and weigh any possible misinterpretations based on commonly held folk or lay beliefs. After you have thought through all possibilities, use metadiscourse to guide the audience. Table 6.4 shows an example of metadiscourse in relation to each of the response strategies introduced in the previous suggestion. Italicized (English) and underlined (Chinese) words indicate metadiscourse

Table 6.4 Response strategies and metadiscourse examples

Response strategy	*Metadiscourse example*
Restate and reframe the question	那大家講就是說齁, 就是說這個是不是文字遊戲啦齁 'Mm everybody *said* this is. Uh I *mean*. Is this *a word game* uh?'
Respond directly and with certainty	那另外我們在感染醫學上我們還常用的另外一個感染地點的分類模式就是, 醫院內感染. 或是我們常說這-, 院內感染. 'Mm also in infectious medicine, we often use another classification method in regards to the infection location. Infections inside a hospital, or we often *called* this hospital-acquired infection.'
Admit the unknown and share the known	不太清楚其他國家的那個國籍嘿... 嘿因為泰國的話他們是宣布很清楚嘛，就是說，他們好像是，是陸- 大陸的國籍，中國籍。 'Not clear about the nationalities of other countries' cases, mh … Mh because in the case of Thailand, they *announce* (it) very clearly. *That is*, they seem to be, be main- mainland nationality, Chinese nationality.'
List criteria	齁那, 通常齁它有幾樣的徵兆，齁專業上來講 'Mh uh, usually mh it has several kinds of signs, mh *professionally speaking*'
Apply each criterion immediately	那如果是在國境之內, 得到感染而後來發病的, 那這個我們就叫作本土個案所以這個, 欸沒有sh- sh-欸, 旅遊史的個案我們大家很清楚他就是所謂的本土個案. 'And if the person is infected within national territories, and afterwards the onset of (symptoms) starts, then we *call this* a local case. So this- uh the case had no sh- sh- uh travel history. We- are all very clear that this is a *so-called* local case.'
Enhance credibility	好我想再請我們教授齁來作回答. 'Ok, I think we will again have our professor *answer* this question.'
Reiterate classification	齁所以這個是-並不是一個文字的遊戲. 齁而是對於相關情況的定義不同, 那讓大家能夠更了解. 'Uh so this is- is not *a word game*, uh but is the use of different *definitions* to relevant situations. So everybody can better understand the situation.'

expressions, for example, verbs of saying, 說 'say'; language referents, 文字的遊戲 'a word game'; and operators that relate propositions, 所謂 'so-called.'

These suggestions for updating existing principles of health crisis communication may appear trivial or imperfect because health crisis situations are always volatile and official communication about the situations is largely determined by individuals' leadership styles. Indeed, no one-size-fits-all approach to health crisis communication can do it justice. However, it is not my intention to overthrow the established consensus about effective communication in public health. In fact, some of the suggestions retain the fingerprints of previous research and existing guidelines. Rather, these suggestions build on the existing wisdom to expand the focus on communicative content to include linguistic and multimodal features that can be used in constructing, circulating, and receiving public health messages.

References

Bauman, R. (2018). Others' words, others' voices: The making of a linguistic anthropologist. *Annual Review of Anthropology*, *47*(1), 1–16. https://doi.org/10.1146/annurev-anthro-102317-045726

Bauman, R., & Briggs, C. L. (1990). Poetics and performance as critical perspectives on language and social life. *Annual Review of Anthropology*, *19*, 59–88. https://doi.org/10.1146/annurev.an.19.100190.000423

Billig, M. (1985). Prejudice, categorization and particularization: From a perceptual to a rhetorical approach. *European Journal of Social Psychology*, *15*(1), 79–103. https://doi.org/10.1002/ejsp.2420150107

Bowker, G. C., & Star, S. L. (1999). *Sorting things out: Classification and its consequences.* MIT Press.

Chang, J.-H. (2021). Invisible storms in the goldfish bowl: Challenges and tactics of journalism under CECC's live press conferences [Unpublished master's thesis]. National Taiwan University. https://doi.org/10.6342/NTU202104411

Dentith, M. (2014). *The philosophy of conspiracy theories.* Palgrave Macmillan. https://doi.org/10.1057/9781137363169

Deschrijver, C. (2024). News media's epistemological framings of the Covid-19 'lab leak' hypothesis: A contrastive metapragmatic analysis of 'conspiracy theory.' In C. Ilie (Ed.), *Manufacturing dissent: Manipulation and counter-manipulation in times of crisis* (pp. 215–239). John Benjamins. https://doi.org/10.1075/pbns.339.07des

Global Views Monthly. (2021, February 23). 新冠疫苗將抵台，你打或不打？《遠見》調查：僅六成民眾願接種 [COVID-19 vaccines are arriving in Taiwan. Will you get vaccinated or not? Global Views survey: Only 60% of public are willing to get vaccinated]. Global Views Monthly. www.gvm.com.tw/article/77926

Goffman, E. (1981). *Forms of talk.* University of Pennsylvania Press.

Hanne, M. (2022). How we escape capture by the "war" metaphor for Covid-19. *Metaphor and Symbol*, *37*(2), 88–100. https://doi.org/10.1080/10926488.2021.1935261

Harel, T. O., Jameson, J. K., & Maoz, I. (2020). The normalization of hatred: Identity, affective polarization, and dehumanization on Facebook in the context of intractable political conflict. *Social Media + Society*, *6*(2). https://doi.org/10.1177/2056305120913983

Jones, R. H. (2021). The wounded leader: The illness narratives of Boris Johnson and Donald Trump. *Discourse, context & media*, *41*, 100499. https://doi.org/10.1016/j.dcm.2021.100499

Latour, B. (1986). Visualization and cognition: Thinking with eyes and hands. *Knowledge and Society*, *6*, 1–40.

Lee, S.-H. (2024). Crisis classifications in mobility: Reporting the first COVID death in Taiwan. *Discourse Studies*, *26*(2), 242–261. https://doi.org/10.1177/14614456231219741

Lempert, M. (2011). Barack Obama, being sharp: Indexical order in the pragmatics of precision-grip gesture. *Gesture*, *11*(3), 241–270. https://doi.org/10.1075/gest.11.3.01lem

McNeill, D. (2005). *Gesture and thought*. University of Chicago Press.

Olza, I., Koller, V., Ibarretxe-Antuñano, I., Pérez-Sobrino, P., & Semino, E. (2021). The # reframe Covid initiative: From Twitter to society via metaphor. *Metaphor and the Social World*, *11*(1), 98–120. https://doi.org/10.1075/msw.00013.olz

Reynolds, B. (2007). *Crisis and emergency risk communication: Pandemic influenza*. https://stacks.cdc.gov/view/cdc/7037

Sachs, J. D., Karim, S. S. A., Aknin, L., Allen, J., Brosbøl, K., Colombo, F., ... & Michie, S. (2022). The Lancet Commission on lessons for the future from the COVID-19 pandemic. *The Lancet*, *400*(10359), 1224–1280. https://doi.org/10.1016/S0140-6736(22)01585-9

Sun, C.-C. (2023). *An analysis of deliberative democracy and political polarization in social media dialogue: A case of YouTube live chat messages on CDC COVID-19 pandemic press conference* [Unpublished master's thesis]. National Taiwan University. https://doi.org/10.6342/NTU202300737

Taiwan Centers for Disease Control. (2020). *Preparedness and contingency planning in response to COVID-19 epidemic*. www.cdc.gov.tw/File/Get/JFnBQLuyGNcuROKLUMjuhA

Tennent, E., & Grattan, F. (2023). The anatomy of a conspiracy theory in Covid-19 political commentary. *Language in Society*, *52*(4), 691–712. https://doi.org/10.1017/S0047404522000197

Tumpey, A. J., Daigle, D., & Nowak, G. (2019). Communicating during an outbreak or public health investigation. In S. A. Rasmussen & R. A. Goodman (Eds.), *The CDC field epidemiology manual* (pp. 243–260). Oxford University Press. https://doi.org/10.1093/oso/9780190933692.001.0001

Wei, T. (2020). The "journalism complication" for Covid-19: A new triangular relationship between the media, the government, and the people. *Taiwan: A Radical Quarterly in Social Studies*, *17*, 199–215. www.airitilibrary.com/Article/Detail?DocID=10219528-202012-202201180006-202201180006-199-215

Wodak, R. (2021). Crisis communication and crisis management during COVID-19. *Global Discourse*, *11*(3), 329–353. https://doi.org/10.1332/204378921X16100431230102

Index

Made in the USA
Las Vegas, NV
19 September 2026

9bf66b6a-a6ad-4467-abd3-b36e39c5aa64R01